How Toxic Are You

How Toxic Are You?

Research clearly proves that our bodies are not capable of eliminating all the different toxins and chemicals we inhale and ingest every day. What can we do?

Benita and Jim Babeckis

Published for:
TRANZFORMATIONS
8571 N. Calle Tioga
Oro Valley, Az. 85704

Email: Tranzform@Comcast.net
Website: http:// Tranzformations.net

Published for Tranzformations
8571 N. Calle Tioga
Oro Valley, Arizona 85704

ISBN 978-1440425592

Type composition and design by Full Moon Rising.

Cover illustration by Jim Babeckis -

Graphic Design and Illustration. Copyright © 2007. Cover design by Full Moon Rising.

First Published October, 2008

Manufactured in the United States of America

How Toxic Are You?

Research clearly proves that our bodies are not capable of eliminating all the different toxins and chemicals we inhale and ingest every day. What can we do?

Benita and Jim Babeckis

Published for:
TRANZFORMATIONS
8571 N. Calle Tioga
Oro Valley, Az. 85704

Email: Tranzform@Comcast.net
Website: http:// Tranzformations.net

Published for Tranzformations
8571 N. Calle Tioga
Oro Valley, Arizona 85704

ISBN 978-1440425592

Type composition and design by Full Moon Rising.

Cover illustration by Jim Babeckis -

Graphic Design and Illustration. Copyright © 2007. Cover design by Full Moon Rising.

First Published October, 2008

Manufactured in the United States of America

Contents

Acknowledgment

This book has been written as a guide for our detox clients and those purchasing detox equipment from us.

Introduction

We are all exposed to thousands of toxins and chemicals on a daily basis at work, at home, in the air we breathe, in our food and water supply, and through the use of pharmaceutical drugs. In addition, we are eating more sugar and processed foods (with less nutrition) than ever before in human history and regularly abuse our bodies with various stimulants and sedatives.

If you never wondered nor cared much about the pollution around us, it's time to change your views (it could be killing you) and start paying attention.

For decades, scientists have been studying the pollutants in our air, water, food, and soil. U.S. industries manufacture over six trillion pounds of 9,000 different chemicals a year. They dump billions of pounds of industrial chemicals into our air and water year after year. So now scientists have started to examine pollution levels in humans and their findings are deeply disturbing.

Research clearly proves that our bodies are not capable of eliminating all the different toxins and chemicals we inhale and ingest every day (http://healthhopeinstitute.com/).

What happens to these toxins?

They simply accumulate in our cells (especially fat cells), tissues, blood, organs (such as the colon, liver and brain) and remain stored for an indefinite length of time causing all kinds of health problems.

How can you help your immune system, improve your health, lose weight, feel better and have more energy? By getting rid of the toxins. How do you do that? Read on.

Chapter One:

Our Toxic World

In this modern, toxic world it's becoming a simple fact of life that our body and all our organs, also requires regular detoxing. Just like a car requires an oil change periodically to clean the engine and remove sludge, so do we.

The "sludge" in us, as in the car, is a byproduct of the combustion of fuel. But the fuels we burn contain more and more processed chemicals and less real nutrition.

How do you know when it's time to free your body of accumulated toxins and other waste materials? If you experience one or more of the following, then it's time to detoxify:

- Candida infection
- Frequent colds
- Excess weight

- Frequent fatigue and low energy
- Impaired digestion
- Irritability and mood swings
- Bad breath & foul-smelling stool,Flatulence, gas & bloating
- Recurring headaches
- Chronic constipation
- Irritable Bowel Syndrome (IBS)
- Food allergies
- Powerful food cravings
- Skin problems, rashes, etc.
- Metallic taste in mouth
- Hemorrhoids
- Protruding belly ("porch")

Maybe you've already heard about the importance of detoxification, you know it's good for you, and you are searching for the best program available. Or perhaps a friend or relative was singing the praises of Tranzformations and said that you just had to check us out. Whatever they may be, you know your own reasons and questions all too well. And we're here to tell you that your search and suffering are over because we know the answer:

You have to get the toxins out and you have to get them out now!

Toxic chemicals, both naturally occurring and man-made, often get into the human body. We may inhale them, swallow them in contaminated food or water, or in some cases, absorb them through the skin.

The term "toxicity level" refers to the total amount of these chemicals that are present in the human body at a given point in time.

Some chemicals or their breakdown products (metabolites) lodge in our bodies for only a short while before being excreted, but continuous exposure to such chemicals can create a "persistent" toxicity level. Arsenic, for example, is mostly excreted within 72 hours of exposure. Other chemicals, however, are not readily excreted and can remain for years in our blood, adipose (fat) tissue, semen, muscle, bone, brain tissue, or other organs. Chlorinated pesticides, such as DDT, can remain in the body for up to 50 years.

"Scientists estimate that everyone alive today carries within his or her body at least 700 contaminants, most of which have not been well studied" (http://www.chemicalbodyburden.org).

This is true whether we live in a rural or isolated area, in the middle of a large city, or near an industrialized area. Because many chemicals have the ability to attach to dust particles and/or catch air and water currents and travel far from where they are produced or used, the globe is bathed in a chemical soup. It bears repeating that we are exposed to chemicals through the food we eat, the air we breathe, and the water we drink and bathe in. Chemicals often coat the surface of dust particles, which we handle or inhale.

Contaminated dust is an especially common route of exposure for children who frequently put their hands into their mouths without washing them.

We are also exposed to hundreds of chemicals in everyday products we use. Paints and varnishes, gasoline, glues, cosmetics, clothes dry-cleaned with solvents, plastic food containers, and home and garden pesticides are just a few examples.

Another source of exposure is the chemical toxicity level of our mothers. During pregnancy, the chemicals stored in a woman's body have the ability to cross the placenta where they may cause harm. Some chemicals from a mother's body are also mobilized and transferred to the breasts as she produces breast milk. These chemicals are then transferred to the baby during breastfeeding. Despite this, breast milk still remains the best food for babies, as recent studies show, because of its immunological, nutritional and psychological benefits.

It has been known for centuries that chemicals can enter the body and cause detrimental health effects. Since the middle of the 20th century, scientists have been able to detect and measure chemicals in wildlif and humans, sometimes linking these chemicals to health outcomes. For example, in 1944 researchers found residues of DDT in human fat, and in the early 50's, naturalists rightly concluded that DDT was directly responsible for thinning eggshells and declining populations of bald eagles and other birds. In fact, at about the same time, DDT was detected in Antarctic penguins living an extremely long distance from anywhere DDT was being used.

Chemicals can have toxic effects through a variety of mechanisms. For example, sometimes a chemical attacks and damages or kills cells or tissues in the body. Some chemicals attack the genetic material in the nucleus of a cell, causing damage directly to the DNA, which may create an inheritable defect that is passed on to the next generation. This can lead to gene mutations, which can set in motion a sequence of events leading to cancer, birth defects, developmental or reproductive disorders.

Dioxin, a toxic substance formed by burning, interferes with normal development, including the immune system. Fetal exposure to polychlorinated biphenyls (PCBs) is related to behavioral and cognition problems. DDT exposure has been related to women's inability to produce sufficient breast milk. The immune systems of children in some areas of the far north are unable to produce enough antibodies to make vaccinations effective. Since these children and their mothers carry large chemical toxicity levels, a chemical link to this problem is likely.

Fetal exposure to mercury causes attention, memory, and learning problems later in life.

Brain development is also impaired in fetuses and infants exposed to lead.

Developing or immature tissues are far more susceptible to chemical exposures than adult tissues. Development is a time of special vulnerability. It is a time of very rapid replication and differentiation of cells - the latter being an incredibly complex and vulnerable process.This means that the developing fetus, infant, or child may suffer harmful impacts from relatively small exposures that have no measurable impacts on adults. So, for example, fetal exposures to chemicals in amounts that are safe for adults may result in birth defects. For this reason, it is not only the amount of the exposure that is important, but the timing of the exposure.

Of the more than *80,000 chemicals* in commerce, only a small percentage of them have ever been screened for potential health effects, such as cancer, reproductive toxicity, developmental toxicity, or impacts on the immune system. Among the approximately *15,000 tested,* few have been studied enough to correctly estimate potential risks from exposure.

Right about now you are probably thinking that the government has regulations and codes that will protect us, regulations that limit harmful chemicals in your food. And you'd be partially right.

What about all the labeling laws and product labels? To a small extent, they do some good. (How often do you read them?) But, they aren't enough. What you aren't aware of is that current regulations were developed well before the advances in science that discovered that small exposures to chemicals - once considered harmless - are indeed capable of subtle cellular changes. New evidence shows that these subtle changes can raise the risk for birth defects, cancer and other health problems. In addition, the regulations now in place are not designed to look at exposures in the context of the full burden of chemicals we carry. No one is looking at the health effects of the cumulative total. U.S. regulations are the result of long, involved political processes in which special interests exert considerable influence.

Industries with significant financial interest in the continued use of a particular product or chemical have historically been quite successful in limiting regulatory controls.

More information about the chemical toxicity levels of individuals, particularly exposed communities, and national populations could help us make better decisions about which products we want to use, which food we want to consume and what laws need to be in place to protect us.

Chapter Two:

Our Immune System

The immune system is the body's means of protection against microorganisms and other "foreign" substances and is composed of two major parts. One component, B lymphocytes (specialized white blood cells), produces antibodies, which are proteins that attack "foreign" substances and cause them to be removed from the body; this is sometimes called the humeral immune system. The other component consists of special white blood cells called T lymphocytes, which can attack "foreign" substances directly; this is sometimes called the cellular immune system. It takes time for both components of the immune system to develop. The only protections a newborn will have are the antibodies that have transferred from the mother to the baby before birth. Over a lifetime, the immune system develops an extensive library of identified substances and microorganisms that are cataloged as "threat" or "not threat."

Vaccinations utilize this process to add to this library. They expose a person's immune system to weakened or inactivated forms of bacteria and viruses, so that the person's immune system will recognize them and create antibodies that will be ready to protect against the infectious forms of these microorganisms if the person comes in contact with them in the future. Normally, the immune system can distinguish between "self" and "not self" and only attacks those tissues that it recognizes as "not self." This is usually the desired response, but not always. When a person is given an organ transplant, the immune system will correctly recognize the new organ as "not self" (unless it is from an identical twin) and will attack it in a process called rejection.

To prevent rejection, a transplant patient must take drugs that reduce the activity of his or her immune system (immunosuppressant's) for the rest of his or her life.

Retinoic Acid, the hormone form of vitamin A, must be present in our bodies for normal functioning of the immune system and for the protein synthesis processes involved in reproduction. Lack of retinoic acid, characterizes most human autoimmune diseases.

The question is whether these diseases are caused by lack of vitamin A or whether lack of vitamin A is caused by autoimmune disease? It turns out that lack of vitamin A is a precondition for the development of many if not all autoimmune disorders. This leads us to ask, what causes a lack of vitamin A?

There are three reasons for a lack of vitamin A in humans. One reason is genetic, a second is dietary, and the third involves exposure to environmental chemicals. Exposure to any of a wide range of environmental chemicals which include pesticides such as insecticides and herbicides and also non-pesticides such as PCBs and dioxin causes environmental illness in both humans and wildlife.

Environmental illnesses include fibromyalgia, chronic fatigue syndrome, multiple chemical sensitivity, and Gulf War Syndrome. All of these diseases appear to be autoimmune in nature. Characteristically, these illnesses occur 5-10 times more commonly in women than in men. The reason for this is that the same process that regulates the immune system also regulates the reproductive cycles in women. Vitamin A (retinol), and vitamin A hormone (retinoic acid), must be present in our bodies for normal functioning of the immune system and for the protein synthesis processes involved in reproduction.

Some people are born with unusually low levels of vitamin A. These individuals have a high sensitivity to sunlight. They need to wear sunglasses on bright days and when they are driving. Autoimmune diseases appear to occur more often in these individuals than in those more tolerant of bright sunlight, mainly because of the lack of vitamin A. The problem appears to be a lower-than-usual ability to make vitamin A from the retinal ester precursors stored in body fat. Inadequate diet is certainly a major factor in vitamin A deficiency. Many third world populations lack access to animal products that supply vitamin A and vegetables that supply vitamin A precursors. The same may be true in the US as well for individuals eating similar poor diets.

The third reason, exposure to many environmental chemicals, is also associated with development of autoimmune disorders. The reason seems to be that exposure to these chemicals poisons the process of making and transporting vitamin A and vitamin A hormone in our bodies. There are several processes that relate to chemically caused deficiencies in vitamin A.

Chlorinated phenyl chemicals such as dioxin and PCBs are known to poison the carrier protein transferrin which moves thyroid hormones and vitamin A from places where they are made to places where they are needed.

It is probable that chlorinated herbicides such as 2,4-D do the same thing as exposures to chlorinated insecticides such as DDT, many synthetic pyrethroids and some organophosphates such as chlorpyrifos may also be involved. Another way Environmental Contaminants reduce vitamin A is by reducing our ability to make it. This occurs when we are exposed to pesticides that poison cholinesterase and other esterase enzymes. A major function of the other esterase enzymes is to activate vitamin A synthesis by hydrolyzing the retinal ester precursors of the vitamin. When vitamin synthesis is low, there is less vitamin A hormone available to activate the immune system. The result is increased frequency of autoimmune disorders.

Autoimmune disorders are diseases caused by the body producing an inappropriate immune response against its own tissues. Sometimes the immune system will cease to recognize one or more of the body's normal constituents as "self" and will create auto antibodies – antibodies that attack its own cells, tissues, and/or organs. This causes inflammation and damage and it leads to autoimmune disorders. The cause of autoimmune diseases is not fully understood, but it appears that there is an inherited predisposition to develop autoimmune disease in many cases.

In a few types of autoimmune disease (such as rheumatic fever), a bacteria or virus triggers an immune response, and the antibodies or T-cells attack normal cells because they have some part of their structure that resembles a part of the structure of the infecting microorganism.

What are some things I can do to feel better?

If you are living with an autoimmune disease, there are things you can do each day to feel better:

• **Detox your body regularly.** Keep your immune system truly healthy and functioning at its peak. Remove chemicals that inhibit immune function or metabolizing of vitamins and proteins from the foods you eat. Try to get all you need from food, rather than from pills. Eat balanced meals with foods from all food groups. Avoid fatty foods made with white flour or sugar. Avoid processed and prepackaged foods.

• **Get regular exercise** (but be careful not to overdo it). Thirty minutes most days of the week is best, but talk with your doctor about what types of exercise you can do. A gradual and gentle exercise program often works well for people with long-lasting muscle and joint pain. Some types of yoga or tai chi exercises may also be helpful.

•   **Get enough rest.** Rest allows your bodies tissues and joints the time they need to repair themselves. Sleeping is a great way you can help both your body and mind. If you don't get enough sleep, your stress level and your symptoms could get worse. You also can't fight off sickness as well when sleep deprived. With enough sleep, you can tackle your problems better and lower your risk for illness. Try to get at least seven hours of sleep every night.

•   **Reduce stress and try "self" pain management.** You may be able to lessen your pain or muscle spasms and deal with other aspects of living with your disease through meditation or self-hypnosis. You can learn to do these through self-help books, tapes, or with the help of an instructor. You also can use imagery (e.g. the power of your thoughts to "destroy" your pain) or distract your focus from the pain by engaging in a hobby or something else you enjoy.

Chapter Three:

Toxins in Everyday Food

While we usually think of toxic substances as coming from man-made sources, many occur naturally. For example, toxic mussel outbreaks in the ocean have claimed lives and caused illness because the mussels consumed contained an algal toxin. Fresh water is not without toxic substances, either. For example, a group of fairly common organisms called cyanobacteria produce toxins called microcystins. The death of cattle, wildlife, and family pets has been traced to drinking water containing microcystins, as have several liver-related illnesses in humans.

Although naturally occurring toxins are all around us, if one is educated to where and how they occur, steps can be taken to avoid them.

Cholinesterase inhibitors

Acetylcholine is a neurotransmitter (a chemical which transmits nerve impulses or signals) in the brain and the peripheral nervous system. The enzyme cholinesterase functions to break down acetylcholine. When cholinesterase is inhibited, the continued presence of acetylcholine over-stimulates the post-synaptic nerve cell, causing the symptoms of poisoning that characterize the anti-cholinesterases. Synthetic insecticides in the organophosphate and carbonate group have the same mechanism of action.

Glyco alkaloids are naturally-occurring anti-cholinesterases, the most common of which are solanine and chaconine. These occur in plants of the genus Solanum, which includes potatoes, tomatoes, and eggplants. The total glyco alkaloid content in potato tubers varies with the variety, with the greatest concentration occurring in the sprouts, peelings, and sun-greened areas.

Poisoning has resulted from ingestion of potato sprouts, sprouted potatoes, and greened potatoes. Symptoms of green potato poisoning include stomach pain, nausea, and vomiting, rapid and difficult respiration, and death. Glyco alkaloid levels of over 20 mg per 100 gram of fresh tissue are considered unsafe. Cooked potatoes with elevated glycol-alkaloid levels have been associated with a bitter flavor, levels higher than 11 mg per 100g could be perceived by some individuals.

Note however, the flavor is not necessarily an indicator of toxicity, nor is the absence of a flavor an indication of a lack of glycol-alkaloids.

Protease inhibitors

Protease inhibitors interfere with the action of trypsin and chymostrypsin, enzymes produced by the pancreas to break down ingested proteins. They are found to some extent in cereal grains (oats, barley, and maize), Brussels sprouts, onion, beetroot, wheat, finger millet, and peanuts. They have caused pancreatic hypertrophy in chicks and rats, but no ill effects have been observed in calves, pigs and dogs.

Trypsin Inhibitors

Raw soybeans have high levels of trypsin inhibitors. Soybean fractions high in trypsin inhibitors depressed the growth of rats, chicks, and mice. Cooking heat largely destroys the trypsin inhibitors in soybeans, but 5 to 20% of the original trypsin inhibitor activity may be retained in commercially available soybean food products. For example, while raw soy flour contains 52.1 TI (trypsin inhibitor activity) per gram of sample, toasted soy flour contains 3.2-7.9 TI per gram.

Amylase inhibitors

Wheat contains a group of anti-enzymes capable of inhibiting amylase, an enzyme present in saliva and the intestinal tract which breaks down starch. Although wheat is rarely eaten raw, and heat destroys anti-amylases, anti-amylase has been found in the center of loaves of bread and in some wheat-based breakfast cereals. Animal experiments and human trials have shown no effect, but could, like protease inhibitors, produce pancreatic hypertrophy if present in large enough quantities.

Tannins

Tannins are present in tea, coffee, cocoa and sorghums. Experimentally they have been shown to interfere with digestibility of proteins, but there is no evidence that they produce an adverse effect in humans. (Tannins have been found to be carcinogenic when injected in experimental animals.)

Cyanogenic glycosides

Cyanogenic glycosides are present in a number of food plants and seeds. Hydrogen cyanide is released from the cyanogenic glycosides when fresh plant material is macerated as in chewing, which allows enzymes and cyanogenic glycosides to come together, releasing hydrogen cyanide. Cyanide is one of the most potent, rapidly acting, poisons known to man.

**Food Sources of Cyanogenic Glycosides and
Amount of hydrogen cyanide (HCN) Produced**

Bitter almonds	250	Amygdaline
Whole sorghum	250	Dhurrin
Lima beans	10-312	Linamarin

Cyanides inhibit the oxidative processes of cells causing them to die very quickly. Because the body rapidly detoxifies cyanide, an adult human can withstand 50-60 ppm for an hour without serious consequences. However, exposure to concentrations of 200-500 ppm for 30 minutes is usually fatal. Acute cyanide toxicity at small doses can cause headache, tightness in throat and chest, and muscle weakness. The effects of chronic (long-term) exposure to cyanide are less well known.

Cooking and other methods of food preparation of green plants before eating can have the effect of diminishing or destroying the natural toxins that exist in the plant material.

Raw soybeans, which often can have high levels of trypsin inhibitors, are seldom eaten without being cooked or heated in some way. Heating destroys most of the trypsin inhibitors in the soybeans, otherwise the proteins in the soybeans would not be available for absorption by the body.

Goitrogens (glucosinolates)

Food plants species in the Cruciferae (Brassicaceae) family contain substances called glucosinolates, which probably play a role in the plant's defenses against predators and fungal attack. However, when eaten by animals or humans, glucosinolates can inhibit thyroid gland functioning, causing enlargement and atrophy of the thyroid, or goiter. Brassica species containing goitrogens include cabbage, broccoli, cauliflower, rutabaga, kohlrabi, and the oilseeds, rapeseed and canola. The enzymes required for production of goitrogens in the plant are destroyed by cooking. Goitrogens are also lost through leaching into cooking water.

Effects in Animals:

Feeding rapeseed meal with high glucosinolate levels to animals and poultry has been found to induce enlarged thyroids, reduced circulating thyroid hormones, liver, kidney, and adrenal abnormalities, and poor growth and reproductive performance.

Effects in Humans:

One study showed no ill effects when volunteers ingested 40 mg goitrin/day in Brussels sprouts over a 4-week period. Another study showed inhibition of iodine uptake after administration of 50-200 mg of goitrin. Studies in Great Britain estimated an average intake of 76 mg glucosinolate per person per day, with a range of up to 200 mg per day. Whether or how much the consumption of Brassica vegetables contributes to ill health in humans is unknown.

The cause of endemic goiter in certain geographic regions may be the result of the interaction between iodine deficiency and certain food components, such as glucosinolates.

Many nutritional studies have shown that dietary fruits and vegetables, including those in the Brassica group, have a protective effect against certain cancers.

In animal studies, glucosinolates and their breakdown products have inhibited tumor formation, although this anti-carcinogenic effect depends on the study design, the type of cancer being studied, whether other dietary components are present, and the timing of the administration of the glucosinolate compound. In summary, glucosinolates are known to be goitrogenic in animals, but their role in inducing goiter in humans is less clear.

They can be anti-carcinogenic and cancer-promoting, depending on the species and circumstances of administration. In general, dietary vegetables, including Brassica vegetables, are beneficial in cancer prevention.

Phytohemagglutinins (Lectins)

Lectin proteins (phytohemagglutinins) are proteins present in leguminous species that can agglutinate red blood cells in various species of animals. These lectins are in many species of beans, especially red kidney beans and castor beans. Poisoning can occur if those beans are eaten raw or not completely cooked.

Lathyrogens

Lathyrogens, found in legumes such as chick peas and vetch, are derivatives of amino acids that act as metabolic antagonists of glutamic acid, a neurotransmitter in the brain. When lathyrogens are ingested in large amounts by humans or animals, they cause a crippling paralysis of the lower limbs and may result in death.

It must be noted that Lathyrism only occurs on an impoverished diet of vetch, sweet pea, or grass pea and is characterized by bone thinning and leg paralysis.

Pyrrolizidine alkaloids

Pyrrolizidine alkaloids (PA) occur in some range plants eaten by animals. These pyrrolizidine alkaloids may enter the human food supply if cereal crops are contaminated with weeds containing the alkaloids, or in small amounts in the meat and milk of animals ingesting the alkaloid containing plants. Pyrrolizidine alkaloids are also found in some herbal teas and herbal medicine preparations. Human poisonings have occurred as a result of the use of home remedies containing these alkaloids. If ingested in large enough doses, pyrrolizidine alkaloids are toxic to liver cells and cause acute liver disease in humans and animals. Some of these alkaloids are potent mutagens and carcinogens in experimental animals. That being said, the importance of these alkaloids in human carcinogenesis is unclear. Many plants from the Boraginaceae, Compositae, and Leguminosae families are contain well over 100 hepatotoxic pyrrolizidine alkaloids.

Anti-thiamin Compounds

These anti-thiamin compounds have been found in mung beans, rice bran, beets, Brussels sprouts, buckwheat seeds, and some berries. Certain bioflavonoids such as quercetin and rutin have been reported to inactivate thiamin.

Thiaminases have been found in fish and shellfish, but are found only in the viscera which are not normally eaten.

Thiamin, or Vitamin B-1, aids in making energy through the metabolism of carbohydrates and is essential for the normal functioning of the nervous system, muscles and heart. Deficiency of thiamin results in a disease known as beriberi. Symptoms include weakness, loss of appetite, irritability, nervous tingling throughout the body, poor arm and leg coordination, and muscle pain deep in the calves.

Avidin

Avidin is a protein present in raw egg white which binds biotin. Biotin (Vitamin B-6) is required for cell growth and for the production of fatty acids. Biotin also plays a central role in carbohydrate and protein metabolism and is essential for the proper utilization of the other B-complex vitamins. Biotin contributes to healthy skin and hair, and may play a role in preventing hair loss. Consuming raw eggs in large amounts over a prolonged period can contribute to biotin deficiency. This is not a problem when consuming cooked eggs, which are a good dietary source of biotin.

Some symptoms of biotin deficiency are depression, lethargy, eczema, dermatitis, anorexia, nausea, vomiting, inflammation of the tongue, and muscle pain.

Chapter Four:

Toxins, Nutrition and Stress

A surprising amount of the stress we experience on a daily basis can be caused by the chemicals we consume. By eating or drinking certain things we can actually put our bodies under chemical stress.

Improper Diet:

At the heart of many of today's illnesses lies poor diet. A healthy diet should include a fresh supply of fruits, vegetables, whole grains, seeds, and nuts, along with poultry and fish. A daily diet of these items would provide all the nutrients our bodies require. Most people today eat unhealthy levels of fat, preservatives, chemical additives, antibiotics and hormones. What, then, is the correct diet for an individual to maintain good health? There are as many "official" opinions about this as there are doctors and every doctor questioned has an opinion and access to research data to support it.

Information on nutritional research is extensive but is often tainted by the social position, politics, or economics of the research organization or their source of financial backing. It is to be noted that while the research into nutrition continues there are still many very old, vigorous, healthy, individuals who smoke and live on food condemned on all sides. These people seemingly live on diets that render laboratory animals sterile, carcinomic, tumor ridden and prone to heart attacks. That these people do live beyond research-set expectations would indicate that no matter how exhaustive the research into nutrition, there are still other factors involved in nutrition that have not been included in any of the research to date. Since there are so very many opinions, as mentioned before, we will not present any of them here, only an overview. Prior to this century, diets were pretty standard, often within a cultural setting. All foods were, what we now call health food - organically grown, unprocessed food, consumed in season. Now, with extensive food processing, most vitamins and minerals are processed out of the food. In place of "real" food, we eat "food products" which may contain, if we're lucky, more food stuff than preservatives.

For a real eye opening experience, read labels.

Although choices abound, and more choices are available, in or out of season due to freezing, drying, canning, dehydrating, homogenizing, concentrating, extruding, and bottling there is less of real value in any of the products despite the advertising claims.

The food processing industry grew out of the need to extend the "selling" life (shelf-life) of products that were being transported, stored and sold cross country from where the actual growing took place.

Ingredients for foods and baked goods are chosen to provide longer shelf life. White flour is capable of being stored longer than wheat or other whole grain flours. Butter with salt as an additive stays "fresh" longer than butter without salt added. Prevention of spoilage is important.

Food can be stored longer and kept for emergencies, it can be shipped across the country and to other countries in times of famine or food shortages. Foods are available in all seasons, providing a wider variety of meal choices for working people.

There is a downside of food processing though, this is the inclusion of chemicals "to retard spoilage," increase "Shelf-Life" as flavor enhancers or to improve texture, smell, or color.

Currently there are over 2,400 additives in use in our food, none of which have to undergo the exacting testing procedures required by the FDA before, let's say, a new drug could be marketed. Although the government regulates the quality and sets sanitation standards for processing plants, enforcement in the food industry is considered by many to be lax at best. Despite ingredient labeling requirements, nutrition is still second to the economic, processing, and marketing needs of producers and distributors in the food industry. With the reliance on processed food, the diet of most of us includes:

- excessive consumption of sugar.
- excessive consumption of salt.
- excessive consumption of preservatives and additives.
- inadequate consumption of fiber.
- inadequate consumption of vitamins and minerals.

Popular health books and nutritional research both agree that specific diseases can be linked to diet. Anyone suffering a long standing illness that is not responding well to traditional medical treatment should consider modifying their diet as a hopeful secondary form of treatment.

Similarly if we are eating an unbalanced diet we may be stressing our bodies by depriving them of essential nutrients.

Eating too much of anything over a long period of time causes obesity. This puts your heart and lungs under stress, overloads your organs and reduces stamina.

• *Caffeine:* Caffeine is a stimulant. One of the reasons you probably drink it is to raise your level of arousal (i.e. stress). If you are drinking many cups of coffee a day, then you may find that you can reduce a lot of stress by switching to good decaffeinated coffee for a portion of your daily intake.

You should be aware of the effects of the following:

• Alcohol: In small amounts alcohol may help you relax. In larger amounts it may increase stress as it disrupts sleep (and causes hangovers!). In large amounts over a long term alcohol will damage your body.

• *Nicotine:* While in the very short term nicotine can cause relaxation, its toxic effects raise the heart rate and stress the body. If you smoke, try taking your pulse before and after a cigarette, and notice the difference. After the initial period of giving up smoking, most ex-smokers report feeling much more relaxed on a general basis. If you are ready to give up smoking, then an excellent book to read is Alan Carr's 'Easy Way to Give Up Smoking'.

• *Sugar:* Sugar-rich foods can raise energy in the short term.

The problem with this is that your body copes with high levels of sugar by secreting insulin, which reduces the amount of sugar in your blood stream. Insulin can persist and continue acting after it has normalized levels of blood sugar. This can cause an energy dip.

If you eat a good, well-balanced diet then you should be able to minimize this sort of chemical stress. Your body will be receiving all the nutrients it requires to function effectively. As with exercise, there is a lot of bad advice on diet available.

If you want to see where you stand, fill out the next two pages. It may surprise you.

1. My Daily Diet

List the foods that you normally eat in any given day. Break these down by meal.

How balanced are your daily meals?

Breakfast:

_____

_____

_____

_____

Lunch:

_____

_____

_____

_____

Dinner:

_____

_____

_____

_____

Caffeine is an ingredient found in coffee, black tea and sodas.

2. How many servings (cups + cans) of caffeine do you drink in a day?

——————— Cups of Coffee

——————— Cups of Black Tea

——————— Cans of Pop

——————— Total

3. Would cutting back help you feel less stressed?

Chapter Five:

Food Additives

Shopping was easy back when most food came from farms. Now, factory-created foods have made chemical additives a significant part of our diet. Most people may not be able to pronounce the names of many of these chemicals, but they still want to know what the chemicals do, which ones are safe and which are poorly tested or possibly dangerous.

A simple, general rule about additives is to avoid sodium nitrite, saccharin, caffeine, olestra, acesulfame K, and artificial coloring. Not only are they among the most questionable additives, but they are used primarily in foods of low nutritional value.

And, don't forget the two most familiar additives: sugar and salt. They may pose the greatest risk because we consume so much of them. Fortunately, most additives are safe and some may even increase the nutritional value of food.

> The Delaney Clause is an important part of the federal Food, Drug, and Cosmetic Act. This important consumer-protection clause specifically bans any additive that "is found to induce cancer when ingested by man or animal." Food and chemical industries are seeking to weaken or repeal that law.
>
> (Annual Review of Public Health, 1997, 18:313-40)

1,1,2-Trichlorotrifluoroethane - Extraction Solvent

The following Health Warnings are about 1,1,2-Trichlorotrifluoroethane were found on the internet at h t t p : / / w w w . c a m d . l s u . e d u / m s d s / t / 112trichlorotrifluoroethane.htm #

Toxicity: Check this out for yourself. Copy any of the additives listed and paste them into your search engine – and we actually consume this stuff! Know what it is that you are eating.

WARNING!

Inhalation: If inhaled, remove to fresh air. If not breathing, give artificial respiration. If breathing is difficult, give oxygen.

Skin: Immediately flush skin with copious amounts of water for at least 15 minutes while removing contaminated clothing and shoes.

Eyes: Immediately flush eyes with copious amounts of water for at least 15 minutes.

Ingestion: Wash out mouth with water provided person is conscious. Call a physician.

1,3-Butylene Glycol - Flavoring Adjunct or Adjuvant, Solubilizer, Solvent, Vehicle

1-Decanol, Natural - Flavoring Agent

Hazards Identification

Emergency Overview

WARNING! HARMFUL IF SWALLOWED OR INHALED. CAUSES SEVERE EYE IRRITATION AND SKIN IRRITATION. CAUSES RESPIRATORY TRACT IRRITATION. COMBUSTIBLE LIQUID AND VAPOR.

SAF-T-DATA(tm) Ratings (Provided here for your convenience)

Health Rating: 2 - Moderate

Flammability Rating: 2 - Moderate

Reactivity Rating: 1 - Slight

Contact Rating: 3 - Severe

Lab Protective Equip: GOGGLES & SHIELD; LAB COAT AND APRON; VENT HOOD; PROPER GLOVES; CLASS B EXTINGUISHER

Storage Color Code: Red (Flammable)

Potential Health Effects

Inhalation:
Inhalation of vapors irritates the respiratory tract and mucous membranes. Symptoms may include headache, dizziness, and other central nervous system effects.

Ingestion:
Low oral toxicity. Small amounts of liquid aspirated into the respiratory system during ingestion, or from vomiting, may cause bronchiopneumonia or pulmonary edema.

Skin Contact:
A skin irritant. Prolonged skin contact may cause dermatitis.

Eye Contact:
An eye irritant. Will injure eye tissue if not removed promptly.

Chronic Exposure:
No information found.

Aggravation of Pre-existing Conditions:
Persons with pre-existing skin disorders or impaired respiratory function may be more susceptible to the effects of the substance.

This is a Flavoring Agent – Oh Yumm! And many other additives feature similar warnings.

1-Octanol, Natural - Flavoring Agent

1-Octen-3-Yl Acetate - Flavoring Agent

1-Octen-3-Yl Butyrate - Flavoring Agent

10-Undecenal - Flavoring Agent

2,3,5,6-Tetramethylpyrazine - Flavoring Agent

2,3,5-Trimethylpyrazine - Flavoring Agent

2,3-Dimethylpyrazine - Flavoring Agent

2,3-Pentanedione - Flavoring Agent

2,4,5-Trimethylpyrazine -3-Oxazoline –
Flavoring Agent

2,5-Dimethylpyrazine - Flavoring Agent

2,5-Dimethypyrrole - Flavoring Agent

2,6-Dimethyl-5-Heptenal - Flavoring Agent

2,6-Dimethylpyrazine - Flavoring Agent

2-Acetylpyrrole - Flavoring Agent

2-Ethyl Fenchol - Flavoring Agent

2-Ethyl-3,5(6)-Dimethylpyrazine - Flavoring
Agent

2-Ethyl-3-Methylpyrazine - Flavoring Agent

2-Ethylbutyraldehyde - Flavoring Agent

2-Ethylbutyric Acid - Flavoring Agent

2-Heptanone - Flavoring Agent

2-Methoxy-3(5)-Methylpyrazine - Flavoring Agent

2-Methoxypyrazine - Flavoring Agent

2-Methylbutyl Isovalerate - Flavoring Agent

2-Methylundecanal - Flavoring Agent

2-Nitropropane - Extraction Solvent

2-Pentanone - Flavoring Agent

2-Phenethyl-2-Methylbutyrate - Flavoring Agent

2-Phenylpropionaldehyde - Flavoring Agent

2-Phenylpropionaldehyde Dimethyl Acetal – Flavoring Agent

2-Triidecenal - Flavoring Agent

2-Undecenol - Flavoring Agent

20 Butanone - Flavoring Agent

3,7-Dimethyl-1-Octanol - Flavoring Agent

3-Acetyl-2,5-Dimethyl Furan - Flavoring Agent

3-Heptanone - Flavoring Agent

3-Octanol - Flavoring Agent

3-Octyl Acetate - Flavoring Agent

3-Phenyl-1-Propanol - Flavoring Agent

3-Phenylpropionaldehyde - Flavoring Agent

3-Phenylpropyl Acetate - Flavoring Agent

4'-Methyl Acetophenone - Flavoring Agent

4-Methyl-2-Pentanone - Flavoring Agent

5'-Guanylic Acid - Flavor Enhancer, Intensifier

5'-Inosinic Acid - Flavor Enhancer, Intensifier

5-Methyl-2-Isopropyl-2-Hexenal - Flavoring Agent

6-Hydroxy-3,7-Dimethyloctanoic Acid Lactone
– Flavoring Agent

6-Methyl Coumarin - Flavoring Agent

6-Methyl-5-Hepten-2-One - Flavoring Agent

Are these all of the additives? Of Course not. There are approximately 2, 400 of them. Benita and I have tracked down and found about 1,100. We only present a few in this chapter. The rest are still unidentified, at least by us, and probably by most people. For the most complete list that we could put together, see Appendix "A" at the back of the book.

Chapter Six :

Our Contaminated Water

The safety of our drinking water is often taken for granted in America, However, in recent years, environmentalists and the media have drawn attention to the dangers of ground water pollution and the health risks of lead, chlorine, pesticides, organic chemicals, and various microorganisms that have been found to contaminate our public water supplies. Outbreaks of waterborne diseases are a common occurrence and have involved entire city populations, sometimes leading to serious complications and even fatalities. The potential carcinogenic effects of long-term exposure to certain organic chemicals in our water supplies are under government scrutiny (http://nepis.epa.gov/) .

Microorganisms: Viruses, Bacteria, and Parasites

Some microorganisms persist as cysts, e.g. Entamoeba histolytica. Asymptomatic cyst carriers are a major source of infection.

Cysts are resistant to disinfectants and they can survive for weeks or months in a moist environment. The prevalence of infection is as high as 50 percent in underdeveloped countries and 5 percent in the United States. Overcrowding and poor sanitation and hygiene have resulted in major waterborne outbreaks, including the Chicago Exposition in 1933, and the Singer Sewing Machine Plant in Indiana in 1950.

The testing of water samples for viruses takes a minimum of two weeks and the tests are not completely reliable.

Bacteriological monitoring is used as the conventional indicator of potable water safety, but viruses are more resistant to water treatment processes than bacteria and may escape detection. Enteric viruses may be present in drinking water without signs of bacterial pollution.

The recycling of waste water for domestic use, now employed in some states with water shortages, may increase the risk of virus contamination. One large beer producer in Southern California, with serious doubts about the purity of the reclaimed water used in the manufacture of its product, has filed a lawsuit in Los Angeles to stop the practice of recycling sewer water. Since 80 percent of beer is water, breweries may have to conduct their own tests for viral, bacterial, and parasitic, as well as chemical contamination, so that jokes about "beer made from waste water" can be dispelled.

Parasites are the most frequently identified cause of waterborne diseases in the United States. The 1993 outbreak of the parasite Cryptosporidium affected almost half a million people and contributed to one hundred deaths in Milwaukee, Wisconsin. The outbreak resulted from the failure of the municipal filtration systems to eliminate animal wastes. In this instance, the water rather suddenly became brownish. Cautious people would have immediately sought out bottled water. Savvy doctors warn people to be alert to changes in their water—either flavor or appearance.

Bottled Water

Concerns about bottled water include the fact that government regulations regarding bottled water are often less stringent than those for public water systems. Bottled water is controlled by the Food and Drug Administration (FDA) and Public water systems by the Environmental Protection Agency (EPA). Their regulations (and the interpretation) can differ somewhat.

Interestingly, one third of all bottled water sold in the United States is actually taken from a public water system. So one must keep in mind that, if the bottled water does come from a deep, protected aquifer, it is less likely to be contaminated than a public water system, that is derived from surface water. "Upland surface water and polluted river sources that have been chlorinated carry the highest risk of cancer. Unchlorinated ground water has the lowest cancer risk" (Nutrition Digest, volume 36, No. 4, 2010).

Even when the water is from an excellent source, storing it in plastic bottles can cause contamination. "It may surprise consumers to realize the enormous potential for risk of intoxication from a multitude of migrant chemicals contained in plastic containers" (J. Gorden Millichap, MD). Government regulation has reduced some of these risks. However, "a carcinogen, methylene chloride, may enter bottled water from the polycarbonate resin in certain plastic bottles, and bacteria may multiply during prolonged storage." (LA Times, June 27, 1986)

Water Treatment Plants: Aluminum and other additives.

In water treatment plants coagulants are employed in order to increase the efficiency of filtration. The use of aluminum and iron salts, sulfates, and polymers in the purification of water may introduce hazards in some individuals, particularly when coagulants are present in high concentration. Aluminum in treated surface water varies widely, and levels higher than 0.2 mg/L cause discoloration.

Water with higher levels may induce encephalopathy [degenerative brain disease] and dementia in patients with kidney disease undergoing dialysis. Aluminum has been linked with Alzheimer's disease.

Air stripping

Air stripping of water, also called aeration, removes some volatile organic compounds (VOCs) such as trichloroethylene and tetrachloroethylene from water by transferring them to the air. It does not remove non-volatile organic chemicals, of equal or greater concern than VOCs.

Radon, a deadly gas, may also be removed from ground water by air stripping but often poses a risk to treatment plant workers, who inhale the contaminated air in the proximity of the aeration system. The inhalation of radon is more toxic than ingestion and the risk of radon-related lung cancer may be increased.

Fluoride

We have to start this section by stating that there is not one single double-blind study to indicate that fluoridation is effective in reducing cavities. (The main reason for introducing a known toxin into our water)

Fluoride is any combination of elements containing the fluoride ion. In its elemental form, fluorine is a pale yellow, highly toxic and corrosive gas. In nature, fluorine is found combined with minerals as fluorides. And yes, it is this chemical that is added to our drinking water. It is the most chemically active nonmetallic element of all the elements and also has the most reactive electro-negative ion.

Because of this extreme reactivity, fluorine is never found in nature as an uncombined element. Fluorine compounds with fluorides are listed by the US Agency for Toxic Substances and Disease Registry (ATSDR) as among the top 20 of 275 substances that pose the most significant threat to human health. In Austrlia, a risk ranking was given based on health and environmental hazard identification and human and environmental exposure to the substance. Some substances were grouped together at the same rank to give a total of 208 ranks. Fluoride compounds were ranked 27th out of the 208 ranks. Fluorides are cumulative toxins.

The fact that fluorides accumulate in the body is the reason that US law requires the Surgeon General to set a Maximum Contaminant Level (MCL) for fluoride content in public water supplies as determined by the EPA. This requirement is specifically aimed at avoiding a condition known as Crippling Skeletal Fluorosis (CSF), a disease thought to progress through three stages.

The Maximum Contaminant Level, designed to prevent only the third and most crippling stage of this disease, is set at 4ppm or 4mg per liter. It is assumed that people will retain half of this amount (2mg), and therefore 4mg per liter is deemed "safe." Yet a daily dose of 2-8mg is known to cause the third crippling stage of CSF. In 1998 EPA scientists, whose job and legal duty it is to set the Maximum Contaminant Level, declared that this 4ppm level was set fraudulently by outside forces in a decision that omitted 90 percent of the data showing the mutagenic properties of fluoride

Mercury

Mercury is discharged into rivers and lakes from many industrial sources such as pulp and paper mills. Mercury itself and some mercury compounds have low toxicity. However, they can be changed into highly toxic "methyl mercury by microorganisms in the water and in the digestive tracts of animals. . . . Methyl mercury penetrates the blood-brain barrier and 10 percent accumulates in the brain, causing irreversible central nervous system damage" (Neuroscience & Biobehavioral Reviews Volume 14, Issue 2, Summer 1990, Pages 169–176).

Methyl mercury accumulates in fish and fish-eating birds and animals. At each step of the food chain there is a bioaccumulation of mercury.

The amount of mercury found in fish may be 3,000 times the original concentration in the contaminated water.

Since methyl mercury is 1,000 times more soluble in fats than in water, it concentrates in muscle and brain tissue. An example of a large scale outbreak of methyl mercury poisoning occurred in Japan in the 1950s when fishermen and their families at Mina Mata Bay were stricken with a mysterious neurological disease. The source of the poisoning was the consumption of fish and shellfish contaminated with methyl mercury derived from materials discharged into the bay from vinyl chloride and acetaldehyde manufacturing plants.

Fish contaminated with mercury from industrial wastes and agricultural insecticides have become a source of concern in the Midwest Inland Lakes of the United States. Recent tests of lake water by the EPA were positive for mercury in 90 percent of samples from 380 different sources in Michigan, Illinois, Indiana, and Wisconsin. At first the symptoms of mercury poisoning are "subtle and diagnosis is difficult. Insomnia, nervousness, tremor, impaired judgment, loss of sexual drive, and depression are symptoms often mistakenly ascribed to psychological causes." Then, "the patient develops a metallic taste in his or her mouth, abdominal cramps, diarrhea, and skin rash."

Later, symptoms from chronic exposure include "a progressive unsteadiness of gait and slurred speech; delusions and hallucinations; and inflammation of the nerves of the extremities associated with loss of sensation, numbness, and pain in the hands and feet."

In the book, *Is Our Water Safe to Drink?,* the author lists preventive measures that include:

- Banning disposal of industrial mercurial wastes in waterways.

- Testing inland lakes and other fisheries for mercury and especially methyl mercury and issue timely warnings and fishing regulations.

- Reducing the mercury content of poultry and seafood which account for nearly all the mercury intake of Americans.

- Eat lake fish sparingly and avoid large trout caught in Lake Michigan.

- Avoid mercury exposure from agricultural chemicals, occupational sources, mercury-containing latex paint, dental amalgams and offices, medicines, thermometers, and household products.

Lead

Lead can be a major drinking water contaminant.

In recent EPA tests of water from household taps, "10 public water suppliers in the State of Illinois, including seven in Chicago suburbs, were included in the list of geographic areas with consumers at risk" (Nutrition Digest, Volume 36, No. 4, 2010).

Many lead pipes are still in use and the solder in joints between new copper pipes often contain some lead. Water that has been standing in the pipes has the highest lead content so people are advised to run their water first thing in the morning until it becomes cold. Where the drinking water is hard -- has a high mineral content -- deposits in the interior of the pipes can seal off much of the lead. For this reason, the water from the taps of new homes and other buildings where lead-containing solder was used in joining the pipes can present even more danger than the water in older homes where the lead has been covered by deposits from hard water. Obviously, water-softening would counteract these helpful effects.

Chlorinated Hydrocarbons

Chlorinated hydrocarbon insecticides are the most widespread and persistent pesticides in the environment. Traces of DDT, one of the more well known clorinated hydrocarbons have been recovered from dust in the atmosphere that has drifted over thousands of miles and contaminated water formed from melted snow in the Antarctic.

DDT and other chlorinated hydrocarbons are fat soluble. They concentrate in the tissues of animals and are transferred along the food chain, killing fish, birds, and mammals. DDT can bioaccumulation in fish to levels more than 10,000 times the concentration in their aquatic habitat. Biological magnification is the term used for this increased concentration of chemicals as they ascend the food chain from small to larger animals.

The levels in human milk may exceed the legal limits permitted in cows' milk. In fact, an analysis of human milk may be the most accurate measure of the extent of contamination of our environment by pesticide residues and other toxic chemicals.

No Simple Answer

Scientists and Toxicologists asked whether or not our water is safe to drink reply that there is no simple "yes" or "no" answer, "given the many variables in water sources, environmental factors, and treatment processes." (http://beforeitsnews.com/health/Tuesday, February 11, 2014)

In regard to cancer from each individual chemical in drinking water, the World Health Organization has set an estimated level that would be linked with one additional case of cancer in a population of 100,000 people over their hypothesized lifetimes of seventy years. Each level is set up for just one chemical and we are subjected to many.

Clearly, there is a risk involved in ingesting low levels of organic chemical contaminants every day of our lives and that one additional case of cancer per 100,000 population might be someone close.

Chapter Seven

Vegetable Oils and Lipid Hydro-Peroxides

Lipid hydro-peroxides, those infamous by-products of vegetable oil processing are the antagonists of our arteries, agitators of our joints, the scourge of our century and an enemy of mankind.

Lipid hydro-peroxides are contaminants that are formed from natural fatty acids when polyunsaturated fats are heated excessively, which happens in processing and when these oils are heated for cooking and frying. Lipid hydro-peroxides poison our body's systems just as trans fats do; in fact, they may even be worse than trans fats because of their propensity to react with oxygen and iron, thereby forming free radicals.

These distortion reactions occur in the factory, the frying pan, and in our bloodstreams. When we eat foods with lipid hydro peroxides, they incite free radical cascades in addition to deactivating enzymes, just like trans fats do.

This makes lipid hydro-peroxides potent toxins, capable of causing tissue inflammation resulting in skin rashes, heartburn, liver problems, arterial spasm and blood clots, and in some cases, even cancer.

Lipid Hydro-Peroxides are strong oxidants in our body and seem to be responsible for producing free radicals, causing damage to the DNA strands within our cells.

Scientific research into the dangers of LHPs is not as extensive as studies into trans-fats, but it is getting some attention now. We can expect more in the future with estimates of health problems these are responsible.

Foods High in LHPs (to avoid)

- Unsaturated Cooking Oils, sunflower, canola, soybean oil etc (especially after used in frying)
- Salad dressings using canola oil and soybean oil
- Most processed foods and supermarket baked goods
- All Margarines (including olive oil and low trans spreads)
- Fried Foods, potato chips, corn chips
- Fast Food fries and chips, cooked in unsaturated vegetable oils*

Foods deep fried in rice-bran oil and or virgin olive oil will not have as high levels of LHPs, but are still not as safe as using Palm oils and high saturated animal fats.

When it comes to knowing which vegetable oil is best and safest to cook with, many restaurants and so-called health experts don't seem to understand basic biochemistry. That's because even the "safe" vegetable oils used by restaurants and recommended by experts convert to seriously damaged breakdown products that have been linked to heart disease and neurological disorders. These include the afore mentioned villan HNE. According to researchers, HNE collects in high amounts in polyunsaturated oils that have linoleic acid, which include:

- Corn
- Canola
- Soybean
- Sunflower

Excessive consumption of vegetable oil can also contribute to:

- Asthma
- Blindness
- Heart disease
- Cancer

This is largely due to the fact that they are highly processed foods and when consumed in massive amounts, as they are by most of us, they seriously distort the important omega-6:3 ratio.

Because of the instability of Omega 3 and 6, consumption of deep fried foods will never be a great source of essential fatty acids, and should never be promoted as such.

A second deadly toxic compound created when cooking with vegitabler oils, has been discovered.

Researchers at the University of Minnesota have identified a highly toxic compound, 4-hydroxy-trans-2-noneal (HNE), which forms in vegetable oils when they are heated to frying temperature (365 degrees) and then concentrate in the fried foods themselves. "HNE is a well known, highly toxic compound that is easily absorbed from the diet," said A. Saari Csallany, professor of food chemistry and nutritional biochemistry at the 96th annual meeting of the American Oil Chemists Society.

"The toxicity arises because the compound is highly reactive with proteins, nucleic acids: DNA, RNA and other biomolecules" (Dr. S. Csallany).

HNE is formed from the oxidation of linoleic acid, and reports have related it to several diseases, including atherosclerosis, stroke, Parkinson's, Alzheimer's, Huntington's and liver diseases."

Consumer's are finding foods with ever higher content of lipid hydro-peroxides due to more added vegetable oil, or to being heated longer, more often, or at higher temperatures. It seems as though vegetable oil is in everything, and everything it's in contains these lipid hydro peroxides, capable of causing almost any disease.

HNE's Effect on the Body

Many studies have linked HNE consumption to increased risks for cardiovascular disease, stroke, Parkinson's disease, Alzheimer's disease, Huntington's disease, liver problems and cancer. Researchers explain that HNE's toxicity stems from the fact that it reacts extremely energetically with biomolecules once it is absorbed into the body by way of our food. Also, it reacts with the various kinds of amino groups--proteins, DNA, RNA adversely affecting basic cellular processes. Unsaturated vegetable oils that are low in anti-oxidants are the most prone to producing these nasties, and they are, per molecule, far more dangerous than any trans-fat molecule! The use of canola oil, sunflower oil and soybean oils for frying has resulted in increasing our exposure to these oxidizing molecules. Now that the use of hydrogenated oils is finally on the decline, we can expect this problem to get much worse

An extreme example can be seen in the fast-food restaurants that are replacing hydrogenated oils with less-refined unsaturated oils, essentially replacing one evil with another, more deadly one! The use of rice-bran oil and virgin olive oils for frying will give some relief from Lipid Hydro-Peroxides, but when oils are used repeatedly, the only safe option is to use stable saturated oils like palm oils and tallow's, and even then regularly replace frying oils.

Making Frying Safe

Use a base oil of beef tallow, coconut oil or palm oil (90%), mix with a small amount of sesame oil (non solvent extracted) for its unique heat-activated anti-oxidants.

High saturated palm oils are the most stable oil, containing already high levels of anti-oxidants (Vitamin E). Palm Kernel oil however is mostly mono-unsaturated and is not as suitable. Beef and lamb fats are the most stable animal fats, being 50-60% saturated, but are not high in anti-oxidants. Pig fat and poultry fats are mostly mono-unsaturated, and are not as suitable.

Coconut oil, with its very high levels of short-chain saturated fats is extremely stable, however by itself it is volatile (evaporates quickly) and is not high in anti-oxidants, so will require some sesame oil to protect the unsaturated components and slow down evaporation.

Chapter Eight:

Sugar or Substitutes

What should you think about artificial sweeteners? We want you to be fully informed about the dangers of Splenda and other artificial sweeteners so that you can make the best choices for yourself and for your family.

Sucralose

"Low–sugar" is the successor to the "low–carb" craze, even though they are essentially the same thing. According to the New York Times, by the end of this summer 11% of the food items on supermarket shelves will be labeled "reduced sugar" — most of those targeted at kids and their health-conscious moms. Sales in granulated sugar have dropped four percent in the past six months. What's behind this trend? Splenda.

Products featuring Splenda are perceived as "natural" because even the FDA's press release about sucralose parrots the claim that "it is made from sugar" — an assertion disputed by the Sugar Association, which is suing Splenda's manufacturer, McNeil Nutritionals.

The FDA has no definition for "natural," so please bear with us for a biochemistry moment: Splenda is the trade name for sucralose, a synthetic compound stumbled upon in 1976 by scientists in Britain seeking a new pesticide formulation. It is true that the Splenda molecule is comprised of sucrose (sugar) — except that three of the hydroxyl groups in the molecule have been replaced by three chlorine atoms. (To get a better picture of what this looks like, check online for the image of a sucralose molecule.)

While some industry experts claim the molecule is similar to table salt or sugar, other independent researchers say it has more in common with pesticides. That's because the bonds holding the carbon and chlorine atoms together are more characteristic of a chlorocarbon than a salt — and most pesticides are chlorocarbons. The premise offered next is that just because something contains chlorine doesn't guarantee that it's toxic. And that is also true, but you and your family may prefer not to serve as test subjects for the latest post-market artificial sweetener experiment — however "unique."

Once it gets to the stomach, sucralose goes largely unrecognized in the body as food — that's why it has no calories. The majority of people don't absorb a significant amount of Splenda in their small intestine — about 15% by some accounts. The irony is that your body tries to clear unrecognizable substances by digesting them, so it's not unlikely that the healthier your gastrointestinal system is, the more you'll absorb the chlorinated molecules of Splenda. So, is Splenda safe? The truth is, it's too early to tell. There are no long-term studies of the side effects of Splenda in humans. The manufacturer's own short-term studies showed that sucralose caused shrunken thymus glands and enlarged livers and kidneys in rodents. But in this case, the FDA decided that because these studies weren't based on human test subjects, they were not conclusive.

People have been using artificial sweeteners for decades. Some react poorly, some don't — the problem is, you never know until you're already sick.

Scientists are calling Splenda a mild mutagen, based on how much is absorbed. Right now, it's anyone's guess what portion of the population is being exposed to the dangers of Splenda or already suffering from Splenda side effects. Until an independent, unbiased research group conducts long-term studies on humans (six months is hardly long-term!), how can we be certain?

With all the new Splenda products on our shelves, it looks as if we are now in the process of another grand public experiment — without our permission. And we may not know the health implications for decades. As with all things, time will unveil truth.

Of course, there are countless examples of foods and drugs that have proved dangerous to humans that were first found to be dangerous to laboratory rats, and then again, countless others that have not. So the reality is that we are the guinea pigs for Splenda.

And now, are our children the next trial group? Thanks to an agreement between McNeil Nutritionals (makers of Splenda) and PTO Today, which provides marketing and fund-raising aid to parents' associations, your elementary school's next bake sale may be sponsored by Splenda — complete with baked goods made with the product.

Observational evidence shows that there are possible side effects from Splenda. These side effects include skin rashes/flushing, panic-like agitation, dizziness and numbness, diarrhea, muscle aches, headaches, intestinal cramping, bladder issues, and stomach pain. These show up at one end of the spectrum — in the people who have an allergy or sensitivity to the sucralose molecule. But no one can say to what degree consuming Splenda affects the rest of us.

If this sounds familiar, it should: we (the U.S.) went down the same path with Aspartame, the main ingredient in Equal and NutraSweet. Almost all of the independent research into Aspartame found dangerous side effects in rodents. The FDA chose not to take these findings into account when it approved Aspartame for public use. Over the course of 15 years, those same side effects increasingly appeared in humans. Not in everyone, of course — but in those who were sensitive to the chemical structure of Aspartame.

Aspartame

Aspartame, the main ingredient in Equal and NutraSweet, is responsible for the most serious cases of poisoning, because the body actually digests it. Aspartame should be avoided by most women, but particularly those with neuropsychiatric concerns.

Recent studies in Europe show that aspartame use can result in an accumulation of formaldehyde in the brain, which can damage your central nervous system and immune system and cause genetic trauma. The FDA admits this is true, but claims the amount is low enough in most that it shouldn't raise concern. We think any amount of formaldehyde in your brain is too much.

Aspartame has had the most complaints of any food additive available to the public (J. Houser, Vanderbilt University, 2005). It's been linked with MS, lupus, Fibromyalgia and other central nervous system disorders. Possible side effects of aspartame include headaches, migraines, panic attacks, dizziness, irritability, nausea, intestinal discomfort, skin rash, and nervousness. Some researchers have linked aspartame with depression and manic episodes. It may also contribute to male infertility.

Saccharin

Saccharin, the first widely available chemical sweetener, is hardly mentioned any more. Better-tasting NutraSweet took its place in almost every diet soda, but saccharin is still an ingredient in some prepared foods, gum, and over-the-counter medicines. Remember those carcinogen warnings on the side of products that contained saccharin? They no longer appear because industry testing showed that saccharin only caused bladder cancer in rats.

Most researchers agree that in sufficient doses, saccharin is carcinogenic in humans. The question is, how do you know how much artificial sweetener your body can tolerate? That being said, some practitioners think saccharin in moderation is the best choice if you must have an artificially sweetened beverage or food product. It's been around a relatively long time and seems to cause fewer problems than aspartame.

We don't argue with this recommendation, but we encourage you to find out as much as you can about any chemical before you ingest it. They are never a good idea for pregnant women, children or teenagers — despite the reduced sugar content — because of possible irreversible cell damage. If you decide it's worth the risks, then go ahead, but pay attention to your body and your cravings.

Once you start tracking your response to artificial sweeteners, it may surprise you. But you should know that sugar substitutes don't have to be artificial. There is another way.

Stevia and Other Polyalcholol Sugars

Other countries and diabetics have both taught us a lot about controlling insulin naturally. For many years, diabetics have used products sweetened with polyalcohol sugars like sorbitol, xylitol, malitol, and mannitol. These are natural sweeteners that do not trigger an insulin reaction. (Xylitol can be derived from birch tree pulp.) They have half the calories of sugar and are not digested by the small intestine.

While most polyalcohol sugars have no side effects, sorbitol is a natural laxative and can cause diarrhea, irritable bowel syndrome, bloating and gas. For this reason and others, we recommend the herb Stevia (Stevia rebaudiana) over sorbitol as a natural sweetener to our friends.

Known in South America as the "sweet herb," Stevia has been used for over 400 years without ill effect. Stevia has been enormously popular in Japan, where it has been in use for more than 20 years, now rivaling Equal and Sweet' N Low. It's 200–300 times sweeter than sugar, so just a small portion of Stevia will sweeten even a strong cup of tea. We've known about Stevia in the US since 1918, but pressure from the sugar import trade blocked its use as a commodity. Today Stevia is slowly gaining steam as a sugar substitute, despite similar hurdles. The FDA has approved its use as a food supplement, but not as a food additive due to a lack of studies.Stevia can be used for anything you might use sugar in, including baking. It is naturally low in carbohydrates. You can buy Stevia at most health food stores and over the Internet.

There will always be those who have a sensitivity to a substance, but based on reports from other countries it appears to have little to no side effects.

For women who want to move through their cravings for sugar without artificial chemicals, Stevia is a great option.

Chapter Nine:

Summary and Solutions

In this book, we've told you a lot about toxins and chemicals that you should avoid, some of which are already processed into our food. We've talked about "dangerous" fats and oils and many other things that are not good for anyone's health. Now it's time to discuss solutions to all of these "problem" areas and find out what you can do to be healthier.

By now, we hope you know that we are exposed to deadly chemicals through the food we eat, the air we breathe, and the water we drink and bathe in. Chemicals often coat the surface of dust particles, which we handle or inhale. Contaminated dust is an especially critical route of exposure for children who commonly put their hands or fingers in their mouths. We are also exposed to hundreds of chemicals in everyday products we use. These products can include: paints and varnishes, gasoline, glues, cosmetics, clothes dry-cleaned with solvents, plastic food containers, and home and garden pesticides, herbicides, weed killers, aluminum in deodorants, peroxide in hair care and hair coloring products, oven cleaners, drain cleaners, roach traps, ant sprays, and cigarettes.

So here's what we know so far: That everyone is exposed to some degree is pretty much a given. Every body probably contains some toxins lodged in their tissues, picked up at some time during their lives. Whether these toxins are hurting them and to what degree, we honestly cannot say. It all depends on body type, age, weight and many other factors. Will you feel better by detoxing and getting the toxins out of your body? Almost certainly. Let's review what has been discovered.

From **Chapter One** we learned that there are over 80,000 toxic substances in use on any given day and only a small percentage of these have ever been tested. Most of those tested have been tested inadequately.

While there are government regulations in place to protect us, most of these regulations were passed before science discovered how even the smallest quantities of toxins can have lasting effects on our system.

In **Chapter Two** we saw how a hormone (retinoic acid), must be present in our bodies for normal functioning of the immune system and for the protein synthesis processes involved in reproduction.

We also saw how lack of retinoic acid, the hormone form of vitamin A, characterizes most human autoimmune diseases.

In *Chapter Three* we learn how naturally occurring toxins are all around us. How many plants that may be consumed by us as raw food or indirectly in cattle can interrupt the functioning of certain enzymes within our bodies. We discuss how hydrogen cyanide is released from the cyanogenic glycosides when fresh plant material is macerated as in chewing, which allows enzymes and cyanogenic glycosides to come together creating the poison. We discuss ways to avoid the naturally occurring poisons by soaking or cooking.

Chapter Four discusses the effects of improper diet on stress and our immune system. This chapter gave us a chance to examine what we eat and discussd how refined sugar, alcohol, nicotine and caffeine impact our stress levels as well as our overall health.

In *Chapter Five* we discuss the 2, 400 + chemicals that are put in food as additives and provided health warnings about several of these that we found.

The entire list of "additives" that we have isolated is too long for the chapter but is provided in Appendix "A."

We encourage each of you to research on your own either at a library or online some if not all of these chemicals and then spread the word to your family and friends.

Everyone should know what is being put in our food under the name of "processing." Avoid processed foods as much as possible.

Read the labels on everything you buy at the super market.

Chapter Six points out the way that toxins such as lead and mercury and other chemicals enter our bodies. We mention several microorganisms that can exist and survive in our water supplies. Chapter Six further warns about some risks involved with bottled water and what to look out for concerning our water.

In **Chapter Seven** we learn about Lipid Hydro peroxides--those nasty, menacing by-products of vegetable oil processing, where they are found and how to avoid them. We have informed you of how researchers at the University of Minnesota have identified a highly toxic compound, 4-hydroxy-trans-2-noneal (HNE), which forms in vegetable oils when they are heated to frying temperatures and what foods to avoid along with how to fry foods safely.

In *Chapter Eight* we discuss the relative value of real sugar and the dangers of the chemical substitutes such as Aspartame, Splenda and Saccharin. We also offer several alternative ways to sweeten tea or coffee. We warn you about the perils of "low-sugar" – "no sugar" products when dieting and the creation of raw sugar or brown sugar from refined sugar.

So what is the root cause of most digestive ailments? It's toxins lodged in the intestinal tract. Just think about what else toxic build-up like this can cause? Stomach pain and constipation? Fatigue, gas and bloating? Headaches and indigestion? Weight gain and a large protruding belly? The list is almost endless. How do you know when it's time to free your body of accumulated toxins, parasites and other waste materials?

If you experience one or more of the following, then it's time to detoxify:

- Frequent fatigue and low energy
- Flatulence, gas & bloating
- Excess weight
- Food allergies
- Impaired digestion
- Irritability, mood swings
- Bad breath & foot odor
- Parasites
- Frequent colds
- Recurring headaches

- Chronic constipation
- Irritable Bowel Syndrome (IBS)
- Protruding belly ("pooch")
- Powerful food cravings
- Skin problems, rashes, etc.
- Metallic taste in mouth
- Hemorrhoids
- Candida infection

In researching this book, we discovered several detox plans on the Internet. We do not endorse any of them. We haven't tried any of them. Most of the plans we ran across involve taking pills of one kind or another. We advise everyone to do your own research. Alternatively, you can ask the person who gave you this book for information on the easiest, safest and most effective plan available.

Let us tell you what we have found . . .

The detoxing Aqua-Chi Foot Spa Units are some of the newest on the market and have already gained popularity due to proven results in helping to purify, cleanse, and detoxify the human body. These units work to deeply rebalance positive and negative ions in your organism and to remove toxins and unwanted waste substances.

Aqua-Chi Foot Spa is a detoxing water bath that cleanses, balances, and enhances the bio-energy present in the body. This energy is the electro-magnetic force that is stored inside the body and is utilized by our cells.

Chinese medicine refers to this energy as "Chi" - a complex energy field that realigns the body's energy while improving the overall condition of the body. While the Aqua-Chi Foot Spa is basically used to increase energy, vitality, and stamina, at the same time it relieves the body from toxins, chemicals, radiation, pollution, synthetics, and other foreign materials trapped in the tissues of the body. This internal cleansing work made possible by Aqua-Chi Foot Spa includes parasite cleansing and liver detoxification, which results in less body fluid retention, reduced inflammation, improved memory, greater bladder control, a more balanced pH, a stronger immune system, and significant pain relief, including the pain of headaches, gout, and arthritis pains.

As noted in Reflexology, each foot of the human body is actually a channel, a conduit, through which our body attempts to cleanse itself of toxic wastes and heavy metals that are building up in many parts of our bodies.

During the Aqua-Chi Footbath session we can actually see the cleansing process taking place, as water interacts with a compound electric current and magnetic field structure. This body cleansing process results in the correct frequency required for the body cells to return to a healthy state, and to release wastes that have been bonded to them over the years.

It is noteworthy that the Aqua-Chi Foot Spa detoxification therapeutic procedure requires no intake of medicine and may also enhance the effects of other therapies.

How the Aqua-Chi® Works

AC electricity is converted to low power DC electricity which flows through a patented electrode system that sits in the footbath. The electricity and the metal combine to split the water molecules into +H and -OH ions. These ions neutralize oppositely charged particles and through powerful osmotic pressure pull those neutralized particles out of the body through whatever skin surface is in contact with the water.

Appendix A:

List of Food Additives and What They Do.

1,1,2-Trichlorotrifluoroethane - **Extraction Solvent**
1,3-Butylene Glycol - **Flavoring Adjunct** or Adjuvant,
Solubilizer, Solvent, Vehicle
1-Decanol, Natural - **Flavoring Agent**
1-Octanol, Natural - **Flavoring Agent**
1-Octen-3-Yl Acetate - **Flavoring Agent**
1-Octen-3-Yl Butyrate - **Flavoring Agent**
10-Undecenal - **Flavoring Agent**
2,3,5,6-Tetramethylpyrazine - **Flavoring Agent**
2,3,5-Trimethylpyrazine - **Flavoring Agent**
2,3-Dimethylpyrazine - **Flavoring Agent**
2,3-Pentanedione - **Flavoring Agent**
2,4,5-Trimethylpyrazine -3-Oxazoline - **Flavoring
Agent**
2,5-Dimethylpyrazine - **Flavoring Agent**
2,5-Dimethypyrrole - **Flavoring Agent**
2,6-Dimethyl-5-Heptenal - **Flavoring Agent**
2,6-Dimethylpyrazine - **Flavoring Agent**
2-Acetylpyrrole - **Flavoring Agent**
2-Ethyl Fenchol - **Flavoring Agent**
2-Ethyl-3,5(6)-Dimethylpyrazine - **Flavoring Agent**

2-Ethyl-3-Methylpyrazine - **Flavoring Agent**
2-Ethylbutyraldehyde - **Flavoring Agent**
2-Ethylbutyric Acid - **Flavoring Agent**
2-Heptanone - **Flavoring Agent**
2-Methoxy-3(5)-Methylpyrazine - **Flavoring Agent**
2-Methoxypyrazine - **Flavoring Agent**
2-Methylbutyl Isovalerate - **Flavoring Agent**
2-Methylundecanal - **Flavoring Agent**
2-Nitropropane - **Extraction Solvent**
2-Pentanone - **Flavoring Agent**
2-Phenethyl-2-Methylbutyrate - **Flavoring Agent**
2-Phenylpropionaldehyde - **Flavoring Agent**
2-Phenylpropionaldehyde Dimethyl Acetal - **Flavoring Agent**
2-Triidecenal - **Flavoring Agent**
2-Undecenol - **Flavoring Agent**
20 Butanone - **Flavoring Agent**
3,7-Dimethyl-1-Octanol - **Flavoring Agent**
3-Acetyl-2,5-Dimethyl Furan - **Flavoring Agent**
3-Acetylpyridine - **Flavoring Agent**
3-Heptanone - **Flavoring Agent**
3-Octanol - **Flavoring Agent**
3-Octyl Acetate - **Flavoring Agent**
3-Phenyl-1-Propanol - **Flavoring Agent**
3-Phenylpropionaldehyde - **Flavoring Agent**
3-Phenylpropyl Acetate - **Flavoring Agent**
4'-Methyl Acetophenone - **Flavoring Agent**
4-Methyl-2-Pentanone - **Flavoring Agent**
5'-Guanylic Acid - Flavor Enhancer, Intensifier
5'-Inosinic Acid - Flavor Enhancer, Intensifier
5-Methyl-2-Isopropyl-2-Hexenal - **Flavoring Agent**
6-Hydroxy-3,7-Dimethyloctanoic Acid Lactone - **Flavoring Agent**
6-Methyl Coumarin - **Flavoring Agent**
6-Methyl-5-Hepten-2-One - **Flavoring Agent**

-A-

Acacia - **Emulsifier**, Foaming Agent, Gelling Agent, Stabilizer, Suspending Agent, **Thickener**, Whipping Agent

Acesulfame Potassium - **Sweetener**

Acetaldehyde - **Flavoring**

Acetanisole - **Flavoring**

Acetic Acid, Glacial - Acidifier, **Flavoring**

Acetic and Fatty Acid Esters of Glycerol - **Emulsifier**, Foaming Agent, **Whipping Agent**

Acetion Acetophenone - **Flavoring**

Acetone - **Extraction Solvent**, Solubilizer, Solvent, Vehicle

Acetone Peroxides - **Bleaching Agent**, Dough Conditioner, Flour Treatment Agent, Maturing Agent, Oxidizing Agent

Acetylated Distarch Adipate - Gelling Agent, **Stabilizer**, Suspending Agent, Thickener

Acetylated Distarch Phosphate - **Emulsifier**, Foaming Agent, Gelling Agent, Thickener, **Whipping Agent**

Acetylated Monoglycerides - Antisticking Agent, Coating Agent, **Emulsifier**, Film Former, Foaming Agent, Glaze, Lubricant, Polish, Release Agent, Solubilizer, Solvent, Surface-Finishing Agent, Texture-Modifying Agent, Texturizer, Vehicle, Whipping Agent

Acid Treated Starch - Binder, Filler, Gelling Agent, Plasticizer, Stabilizer, Suspending Agent, **Thickener**

Activated Carbon - Decolorizing Agent, Odor Removing Agent, Taste Removing Agent

Adipic Acid - Buffer, **Neutralizing Agent**

Agar - **Emulsifier**, Foaming Agent, Gelling Agent, Stabilizer, Suspending Agent, Thickener, Whipping Agent

Alginic Acid - **Emulsifier**, Foaming Agent, Gelling Agent, Stabilizer, Suspending Agent, Thickener, Whipping Agent

Alkaline Treated Starch - Binder, Filler, Gelling Agent, Plasticizer, Stabilizer, Suspending Agent, Thickener

Allura Red Ac - **Color**
Allyl alpha-Ionone - **Flavoring**
Allyl Cyclohexanepropionate - **Flavoring**
Allyl Heptanoate - **Flavoring**
Allyl Hexanoate - **Flavoring**
Allyl Isothiocyanate - **Flavoring**
Allyl Isovalerate - **Flavoring**
Allyl Tiglate - **Flavoring**
Almond Oil, Bitter, FFPA - **Flavoring**
alpha-Amyl Cinnamic Aldehyde - **Flavoring**
alpha-Amyl Cinnamic Aldehyde Dimethyl Acetal -
Flavoring
alpha-Amyl Cinnamyl Alcohol - **Flavoring Agent**
alpha-Amylase (Aspergillus Oryzae) - Enzyme
alpha-Amylase (Bacillus Megaterium) Expressed in
Bacillus Subtilis - Enzyme
alpha-Amylase (Bacillus Stearothermophilus) - Enzyme
alpha-Amylase (Bacillus Stearothermophilus) Expressed
in Bacillus Subtilis - Enzyme
alpha-Amylase (Bacillus Subtilis) - Enzyme
alpha-Amylase and Glucoamylase (Aspergillus Oryzae) -
Enzyme
alpha-Amylcinnamaldehyde - **Flavoring**
alpha-Hexyl Cinnamic Aldehyde - **Flavoring**
alpha-Hexylcinnamaldehyde - **Flavoring**
alpha-Ionone - **Flavoring**
alpha-Methyl Cinnamic Aldehyde - **Flavoring**
alpha-Methylbenzyl Alcohol - **Flavoring**
alpha-Methylcinnamaldehyde - **Flavoring**
alpha-Phellandrene - **Flavoring**
alpha-Pinene - **Flavoring**
alpha-Terpinene - **Flavoring**
Aluminum Ammonium Sulfate - **Color** Fixative,
Firming Agent
Aluminum Potassium Sulfate - Buffer, **Firming Agent**,
Neutralizing Agent

Aluminum Powder - **Color**
Aluminum Silicate - Anticaking Agent, Drying Agent
Aluminum Sodium Sulfate - Buffer, **Firming Agent**, Neutralizing Agent
Aluminum Sulfate - **Firming Agent**
Aluminun Ammonium Sulfate - Buffer, Neutralizing Agent
Amaranth - **Color**
Ambrette Seed Oil - **Flavoring**
Ammonium Adipate - Buffer, Neutralizing Agent
Ammonium Alginate - **Emulsifier**, Foaming Agent, Gelling Agent, Stabilizer, Suspending Agent, Thickener, Whipping Agent
Ammonium Bicarbonate - Alkali, Leavening Agent
Ammonium Carbonate - Buffer, General Purpose Additive, Leavening Agent, Neutralizing Agent
Ammonium Chloride - Dough Conditioner, Yeast Food
Ammonium Dihydrogen Phosphate - Buffer, Dough Conditioner, Leavening Agent, Neutralizing Agent
Ammonium Hydrogen Carbonate - Alkali, Leavening Agent
Ammonium Hydroxide - Alkali
Ammonium Persulfate - Flour Treatment Agent
Ammonium Phosphate, Dibasic - Buffer, Dough Conditioner, Leavening Agent, Neutralizing Agent, Yeast Food
Ammonium Phosphate, Monobasic - Buffer, Dough Conditioner, Leavening Agent, Neutralizing Agent, Yeast Food
Ammonium Saccharin - Nonnutritive Sweetener, Sugar Substitute
Ammonium Salts of Phosphatidic Acid - **Emulsifier**, Foaming Agent, Whipping Agent
Ammonium Sulfate - Dough Conditioner, General Purpose Additive, Yeast Food

Amyl Acetate - Carrier Solvent, Flavoring
Amyl Cinnamate - Flavoring
Amyl Octanoate - Flavoring
Amyl Propionate - Flavoring
Amyloglucosidases (Aspergillus Niger Var.) - Enzyme
Amyris Oil, West Indian Type - Flavoring
Anethole - Flavoring
Angelica Root Oil - Flavoring
Anise Oil - Flavoring
Anisole - Flavoring
Anisyl Acetate - Flavoring
Anisyl Alcohol - Flavoring
Anisylacetone - Flavoring
Annatto Extracts - **Color**
Anoxomer - Antioxidant
Ascorbic Acid - Antioxidant, **Dietary Supplement**, Nutrient, Preservative
Ascorbyl Palmitate - Antioxidant
Ascorbyl Stearate - Antioxidant
Aspartame - Flavor Enhancer, Intensifier, Nonnutritive Sweetener, Sugar Substitute, Sweetener
Avian Pepsin - Enzyme
Azodicarbonamide - Flour Treatment Agent, Maturing Agent
Azorubine - **Color**

-B-
Balsam Peru Oil - **Flavoring Agent**
Basil Oil, Comoros Type - **Flavoring Agent**
Basil Oil, European Type - **Flavoring Agent**
Bay Oil - **Flavoring Agent**
Beeswax, White - Coating Agent, Film Former, **Firming Agent**, General Purpose Additive, Glaze, Polish, Surface-Finishing Agent

Beeswax, Yellow - Coating Agent, Film Former, **Firming Agent**, General Purpose Additive, Glaze, Polish, Surface-Finishing Agent
Beet Red **Color**
Bennzoic Acid - Antimicrobial Agent, Preservative
Benzaldehyde - **Flavoring Agent**
Benzoic Acid - Preservative
Benzoin Gum - **Flavoring Agent**
Benzophenone - **Flavoring Agent**
Benzoyl Peroxide - Bleaching Agent, Oxidizing Agent
Benzyl Acetate - **Flavoring Agent**
Benzyl Bezoate - **Flavoring Agent**
Benzyl Alcohol - Carrier Solvent, **Flavoring Agent**
Benzyl Butyrate - **Flavoring Agent**
Benzyl Cinnamate - **Flavoring Agent**
Benzyl Isobutyl Carbinol - **Flavoring Agent**
Benzyl Isobutyrate - **Flavoring Agent**
Benzyl Isoeugenyl Ether - **Flavoring Agent**
Benzyl Isovalerate - **Flavoring Agent**
Benzyl Phenylacetate - **Flavoring Agent**
Benzyl Propionate - **Flavoring Agent**
Benzyl Salicylate - **Flavoring Agent**
Benzyl Utyl Ether - **Flavoring Agent**
Bergamot Oil, Expressed - **Flavoring Agent**
beta-Apo-8'-Carotenal - **Color**
beta-Apo-8'-Carotenoic Acid, Ethyl Ester - **Color**
beta-Caritebe (Synthetic) - **Color**
beta-Carotene - **Dietary Supplement**, Nutrient
beta-Caryophyllene - **Flavoring Agent**
beta-Glucanase (Aspergillus Niger, Var.) - Enzyme
beta-Glucanase (Trichoderma Harzianum) - Enzyme
beta-Ionone - **Flavoring Agent**
beta-Pinene - **Flavoring Agent**

BHA - Antioxidant
BHT - Antioxidant
Biotin - **Dietary Supplement**, Nutrient
Birch Tar Oil, Rectified - **Flavoring Agent**
Black Pepper Oil - **Flavoring Agent**
Blackcurrant Extract - **Color**
Bleached Starch - Binder, Filler, Gelling Agent, Plasticizer, Stabilizer, Suspending Agent, Thickener
Bois De Rose Oil - **Flavoring Agent**
Bone Phosphate - Anticaking Agent, Drying Agent, **Emulsifier**, Foaming Agent, Humectant, Moisture-Retaining Agent, Whipping Agent
Bornyl Acetate - **Flavoring Agent**
Brilliant Black Pn - **Color**
Brilliant Blue FCF - **Color**
Bromelain - **Enzyme** Brominated Vegetable Oil - Cloud Producing Agent, Flavoring Adjunct or Adjuvant, **Flavoring Agent**, Stabilizer, Suspending Agent
Brown FK - **Color**
Brown HT - **Color**
Butadiene-Styrene 50/50 Rubber - Chewing Gum Base Component
Butadiene-Styrene 75/25 Rubber - Chewing Gum Base Component
Butan-1-Ol - **Extraction Solvent**, Flavoring Agent
Butan-2-Ol - **Extraction Solvent**, Flavoring Agent
Butan-3-One-2-Yl Butyrate - **Flavoring Agent**
Butane-1,3-Diol - Carrier Solvent
Butyl Acetate - **Flavoring Agent**
Butyl Alcohol - **Flavoring Agent**
Butyl Butyrate - **Flavoring Agent**
Butyl Butyryllactate - **Flavoring Agent**
Butyl Isobutyrate - **Flavoring Agent**
Butyl P-Hydroxybenzoate - Antimicrobial Agent, Preservative
Butylated Hydroxyanisole - Antioxidant

Butylated Hydroxymethylphenol - Antioxidant
Butylated Hydroxytoluene - Antioxidant
Butyraldehyde - **Flavoring Agent**
Butyric Acid - **Flavoring Agent**

-C-
Caffeine - **Flavoring Agent**
Calcium 5'-Guanylate - Flavor Enhancer, Intensifier
Calcium 5'-Inosinate - Flavor Enhancer, Intensifier
Calcium 5'-Ribonucleotides - Flavor Enhancer, Intensifier
Calcium Acetate - Antimold Agent, Antirope Agent,
Buffer, Neutralizing Agent, Sequestrant, Stabilizer,
Suspending Agent
Calcium Alginate **Emulsifier**, Foaming Agent, Gelling
Agent, Stabilizer, Suspending Agent, Thickener,
Whipping Agent
Calcium Aluminum Silicate - Anticaking Agent, Drying
Agent
Calcium Ascorbate - Antioxidant
Calcium Benzoate - Antimicrobial Agent, Preservative
Calcium Bromate - Dough Conditioner, Maturing Agent
Calcium Carbonate - Alkali, Anticaking Agent, **Dietary
Supplement**, Dough Conditioner, Drying Agent,
Firming Agent, Nutrient, Yeast Food
Calcium Chloride - **Firming Agent**, General Purpose
Additive, Sequestrant
Calcium Chloride Solution - **Firming Agent**, General
Purpose Additive, Sequestrant
Calcium Chloride, Anhydrous - **Firming Agent**, General
Purpose Additive, Sequestrant
Calcium Citrate - Buffer, **Firming Agent**, Neutralizing
Agent, Sequestrant
Calcium Cyclamates - **Sweetening Agent**
Calcium Di-L-Glutamate - Flavor Enhancer, Intensifier,
Salt Substitute

Calcium Dihydrogen Phosphate - Buffer, **Firming Agent**, Leavening Agent, Neutralizing Agent, Texture-Modifying Agent, Texturizer

Calcium Disodium EDTA - Preservative, Sequestrant

Calcium Disodium Ethylenediamine-Tetraacetate - Antioxidant Synergist, Preservative, Sequestrant

Calcium DL-Malate - Buffer, Neutralizing Agent, Seasoning Agent

Calcium Ferrocyanide - Anticaking Agent, Drying Agent

Calcium Gluconate - Buffer, **Firming Agent**, General Purpose Additive, Neutralizing Agent, Sequestrant

Calcium Glycerophosphate - **Dietary Supplement**, Nutrient Calcium Hydrogen Sulfite - **Firming Agent**, Preservative

Calcium Hydroxide - Buffer, **Firming Agent**, General Purpose Additive, Neutralizing Agent

Calcium Iodate - Dough Conditioner, Flour Treatment Agent

Calcium Lacate - Dough Conditioner

Calcium Lactate - Buffer, Neutralizing Agent, Yeast Food

Calcium Lactobionate - **Firming Agent**

Calcium Monohydrogen Phosphate - Dough Conditioner, Yeast Food

Calcium Oxide - Alkali, **Dietary Supplement**, Dough Conditioner, Nutrient, Yeast Food

Calcium Pantothenate - **Dietary Supplement**, Nutrient

Calcium Pantothenate, Calcium Chloride Double Salt - **Dietary Supplement**, Nutrient

Calcium Pantothenate, Racemic - **Dietary Supplement**, Nutrient

Calcium Peroxide - Bleaching Agent, Dough Conditioner, Flour Treatment Agent, Oxidizing Agent

Calcium Phosphate, Dibasic - **Dietary Supplement**, Dough Conditioner, Nutrient, Yeast Food

Calcium Phosphate, Monobasic - Buffer, **Dietary Supplement**, Dough Conditioner, **Firming Agent**, Leavening Agent, Neutralizing Agent, Nutrient, Sequestrant, Yeast Food

Calcium Phosphate, Tribasic - Anticaking Agent, Buffer, **Dietary Supplement**, Drying Agent, Neutralizing Agent, Nutrient

Calcium Polyphosphates - **Emulsifier**, Foaming Agent, Humectant, Moisture-Retaining Agent, Sequestrant, Texture-Modifying Agent, Texturizer, Whipping Agent

Calcium Propionate - Antimold Agent, Antirope Agent, Preservative

Calcium Pyrophosphate - Buffer, **Dietary Supplement**, Neutralizing Agent, Nutrient

Calcium Saccharin - Nonnutritive Sweetener, Sugar Substitute, **Sweetening Agent**

Calcium Silicate - Anticaking Agent, Drying Agent, Filter Aid

Calcium Sorbate - Antimicrobial Agent, Fungistatic Agent, Preservative

Calcium Stearate - Anticaking Agent, Binder, Drying Agent, **Emulsifier**, Filler, Foaming Agent, Plasticizer, Whipping Agent

Calcium Stearoyl Lactylate - Dough Conditioner, **Emulsifier**, Foaming Agent, Stabilizer, Suspending Agent, Whipping Agent

Calcium Sulfate - **Dietary Supplement**, Dough Conditioner, **Firming Agent**, Nutrient, Sequestrant, Yeast Food

Calciumiodate Maturing Agent

Camphene - **Flavoring Agent**

Cananga Oil - **Flavoring Agent**

Candelilla Wax - Chewing Gum Base Component, Coating Agent, Film Former, Glaze, Polish, Surface-Finishing Agent

Canthaxanthin - **Color**
Caramel Color I (Plain) - **Color**
Caramel Color II (Caustic Sulfite Process) - **Color**
Caramel Colors - **Color**
Caraway Oil - **Flavoring Agent**
Carbohydrase (Aspergillus Nigar Var.
Awamori) - Enzyme
Carbohydrase (Aspergillus Niger Var.) - Enzyme
Carbohydrase (Aspergillus Oryzae Var.) - Enzyme
Carbohydrase (Bacillus Licheniformis) - Enzyme
Carbohydrase (Rhizopus Oryzae Var.) - Enzyme
Carbohydrase (Saccharoomyces Species) - Enzyme
Carbohydrase (Trichoderms Reesei Var.) - Enzyme
Carbohydrase and Protease, Mixed (Bacillus
Licheniformis) - Enzyme
Carbohydrase and Protease, Mixed (Bacillus Subtilis) -
Enzyme
Carbon Dioxide - Carbonating Agent, **Extraction
Solvent**, Packing Gas

-D-
D-alpha-Tocopherol - Antioxidant, **Dietary Supplement**,
Nutrient
D-alpha-Tocopheryl Acetate - **Dietary Supplement**,
Nutrient D-alpha-Tocopheryl Acid Succinate - **Dietary
Supplement**, Nutrient
D-Carvone - **Flavoring Agent**
D-Dihydrocarvone - **Flavoring Agent**
D-Limonene - **Flavoring Agent**
Dammar Gum - Gelling Agent, Stabilizer, Suspending
Agent, Thickener
Decanal - **Flavoring Agent**
Decanoic Acid - Component in the Manufacture of Other
Food-Grade, Additives, Defoaming Agent, **Flavoring
Agent**

Dehydroacetic Acid - Preservative
delta-Decalactone - **Flavoring Agent**
delta-Dodecalactone - **Flavoring Agent**
Desoxycholic Acid - **Emulsifier**, Foaming Agent, Whipping Agent
Dexpanthenol - **Dietary Supplement**, Nutrient
Dextrin - Binder, Filler, Gelling Agent, Plasticizer, Stabilizer, Suspending Agent, Thickener
Dextrin Ethyl Cellulose - Coating Agent, Film Former, Glaze, Polish, Surface-Finishing Agent
Dextrins, Roasted - Starch Binder, Filler, Gelling Agent, Plasticizer, Stabilizer, Suspending Agent, Thickener
Dextrose - Carrier, Disintegrating Agent, Dispersing Agent, Formulation Aid, Humectant, Moisture-Retaining Agent, Nutritive Sweetener, Tableting Aid, Texture-Modifying Agent, Texturizer
Diacetyl - **Flavoring Agent**
Diacetyl Tartaric Acid Esters of Mono- and Diglycerides - **Emulsifier**, Foaming Agent, Whipping Agent
Diacetyltartaric and Fatty Acid Esters of Glycerol - **Emulsifier**, Foaming Agent, Whipping Agent
Diammonium Hydrogen Phosphate - Buffer, Dough Conditioner, Leavening Agent, Neutralizing Agent, Yeast Food
Diatomaceous Earth - **Filter Aid**
Dibenzyl Ether - **Flavoring Agent**
Dibutyl Sebacate - **Flavoring Agent**
Dicalcium Pyrophosphate - Buffer, Neutralizing Agent, Yeast Food
Dichloromethane - **Extraction Solvent**
Diethyl Ether - **Extraction Solvent**
Diethyl Malonate - **Flavoring Agent**
Diethyl Pyrocarbonate - Antimicrobial Agent, Preservative
Diethyl Sebacate - **Flavoring Agent**

Diethyl Succinate - **Flavoring Agent**
Diethyl Tartrate - Carrier Solvent, **Flavoring Agent**
Diethylene Glycol Monoethyl Ether - Carrier Solvent,
Extraction Solvent
Dihydrocarveol - **Flavoring Agent**
Dihydrocoumarin - **Flavoring Agent**
Dilauryl Thiodipropionate - Antioxidant
Dill Seed Oil, European Type - **Flavoring Agent**
Dill Seed Oil, Indian Type - **Flavoring Agent**
Dillweed Oil, American Type - **Flavoring Agent**
Dimethyl Anthranilate - **Flavoring Agent**
Dimethyl Benxyl Carbinyl Acetate - **Flavoring Agent**
Dimethyl Benzyl Carbinol - **Flavoring Agent**
Dimethyl Benzyl Carbinyl - Butyrate **Flavoring Agent**
Dimethyl Dicaronate - Preservative
Dimethylpolysiloxane - Defoaming Agent
Dioctyl Sodium Sulfosuccinate - **Emulsifier**, Foaming
Agent, Surface-Active Agent, Wetting Agent, Whipping
Agent
Diphenyl - Fungistatic Agent
Dipotassium 5'-Guanylate - Flavor Enhancer, Intensifier
Dipotassium 5'-Inosinate - Flavor Enhancer, Intensifier
Dipotassium Hydrogen Phosphate - Buffer, Neutralizing
Agent, Sequestrant, Yeast Food
Disodium 5'-Guanylate - Flavor Enhancer, Intensifier
Disodium 5'-Inosinate - Flavor Enhancer, Intensifier
Disodium 5'-Ribonucleotides - Flavor Enhancer,
Intensifier
Disodium EDTA - Preservative, Sequestrant, Stabilizer,
Suspending Agent
Disodium Ethylenediamine-Tetraacetate - Antioxidant
Synergist, Preservative, Sequestrant
Disodium Guanylate - Flavor Enhancer, Intensifier

Disodium Hydrogen Phosphate - Buffer, **Emulsifier**, Foaming Agent, Neutralizing Agent, Texture-Modifying Agent, Texturizer, Whipping Agent

Disodium Inosinate - Flavor Enhancer, Intensifier

Disodium Pyrophosphate - Buffer, Leavening Agent, Neutralizing Agent, Sequestrant, Stabilizer, Suspending Agent

Distarch Phosphate - Binder, Filler, Gelling Agent, Plasticizer, Stabilizer, Suspending Agent, Thickener

DL-Alanine - **Dietary Supplement**, Nutrient

DL-alpha-Tocopherol - Antioxidant, **Dietary Supplement**, Nutrient

DL-alpha-Tocopheryl Acetate - **Dietary Supplement**, Nutrient

DL-Aspartic Acid - **Dietary Supplement**, Nutrient

DL-Isoleucine - **Dietary Supplement**, Nutrient

DL-Leucine - **Dietary Supplement**, Nutrient

DL-Malic Acid - Acid, Acidifier, **Flavoring Agent**

DL-Menthol - **Flavoring Agent**

DL-Menthyl Acetate - **Flavoring Agent**

DL-Methionine - **Dietary Supplement**, Nutrient

DL-Panthenol - **Dietary Supplement**, Nutrient

DL-Phenylalanine - **Dietary Supplement**, Nutrient

DL-Serine - **Dietary Supplement**, Nutrient

DL-Tartaric Acid - Acid, Acidifier, Antioxidant Synergist, **Emulsifier**, Foaming Agent, Sequestrant, Whipping Agent

DL-Tryptophan - **Dietary Supplement**, Nutrient

Dodecyl Gallate - Antioxidant

-E-

Edible Gelatin - **Emulsifier**, Foaming Agent, Gelling Agent, Stabilizer, Suspending Agent, Whipping Agent

Enzyme Treated Starches - Gelling Agent, Thickener

Erythorbic Acid - Antioxidant, Preservative

Esters of Glycerol and Thermally Oxidized Soy Bean Fatty Acids - Antispattering Agent, **Emulsifier**, Foaming Agent, Whipping Agent

Estragole **Flavoring Agent**

Ethoxylated Mono- and Diglycerides - **Emulsifier**, Foaming Agent, Whipping Agent

Ethoxyquin - Antioxidant

Ethyl 2-Methylbutyrate - **Flavoring Agent**

Ethyl Aacetoacetate - **Flavoring Agent**

Ethyl Acetate - Carrier Solvent, **Flavoring Agent**

Ethyl Acrylate - **Flavoring Agent**

Ethyl Alcohol - Carrier Solvent, **Extraction Solvent**, Solubilizer, Solvent, Vehicle

Ethyl Anthranilate - **Flavoring Agent**

Ethyl Benzoate - **Flavoring Agent**

Ethyl Butyrate - **Flavoring Agent**

Ethyl Cellulose - Binder, Carrier, Dilatants of Color and Food Additives, Disintegrating Agent, Dispersing Agent, Filler, Formulation Aid, Plasticizer, Tableting Aid

Ethyl Cinnamate - **Flavoring Agent**

Ethyl Decanoate - **Flavoring Agent**

Ethyl Formate - **Flavoring Agent**

Ethyl Heptanoate - **Flavoring Agent**

Ethyl Hexanoate - **Flavoring Agent**

Ethyl Hydroxyethyl Cellulose - **Emulsifier**, Foaming Agent, Gelling Agent, Stabilizer, Suspending Agent, Thickener, Whipping Agent

Ethyl Isovalerate - **Flavoring Agent**

Ethyl Lactate - **Flavoring Agent**

Ethyl Laurate - **Flavoring Agent**

Ethyl Maltol - Flavor Enhancer, Intensifier, **Flavoring Agent**

Ethyl Methyl Ketone - **Extraction Solvent, Flavoring Agent**

Ethyl Methylphenylglycidat - **Flavoring Agent**

Ethyl Nonanoate - **Flavoring Agent**
Ethyl Oxyhydrate - **Flavoring Agent**
Ethyl P-Anisate - **Flavoring Agent**
Ethyl P-Hydroxybenzoate - Antimicrobial Agent, Preservative
Ethyl Phenylacetate - **Flavoring Agent**
Ethyl Phenylglycidate - **Flavoring Agent**
Ethyl Propionate - **Flavoring Agent**
Ethyl Protocatechuate - Antioxidant
Ethyl Salicylate - **Flavoring Agent**
Ethyl Vanillin - **Flavoring Agent**
Ethylene Dichloride - Solubilizer, Solvent, Vehicle
Ethylene Oxide - Fumigant
Ethyoxylated Mono- and Diglyerides - Dough Conditioner
Eucalyptol - **Flavoring Agent**
Eucalyptus Oil - **Flavoring Agent**
Eugenol - **Flavoring Agent**
Eugenyl Acetate - **Flavoring Agent**
Eugenyl Methyl Ether - **Flavoring Agent**

-**F**-
Farnesol - **Flavoring Agent**
Fast Green FCF - **Color**
Fast Red E - **Color**
Fennel Oil - **Flavoring Agent**
Ferric Ammonium Citrate - Anticaking Agent, **Dietary Supplement**, Drying Agent, Nutrient
Ferric Phosphate - **Dietary Supplement**, Nutrient
Ferric Pyrophosphate - **Dietary Supplement**
Ferrous Ammonium Citrate, Brown - **Dietary Supplement**, Nutrient
Ferrous Ammonium Citrate, Green - Anticaking Agent, **Dietary Supplement**, Drying Agent, Nutrient
Ferrous Fumarate - **Dietary Supplement**, Nutrient
Ferrous Gluconate - Color Adjunct, **Dietary Supplement**, Nutrient

Ferrous Lactate - **Color Adjunct**
Ferrous Sulfate - **Dietary Supplement**, Nutrient
Ferrous Sulfate, Dried - **Dietary Supplement**, Nutrient
Ficin - Enzyme
Fir Needle Oil, Canadian Type - **Flavoring Agent**
Fir Needle Oil, Siberian Type - **Flavoring Agent**
Folic Acid - **Dietary Supplement**, Nutrient
Food Starch, Modified - **Binder**, Filler, Gelling Agent,
Plasticizer, Stabilizer, Suspending Agent, Thickener
Formic Acid - **Flavoring Adjunct** or Adjuvant,
Preservative
Fructose - Carrier, **Disintegrating Agent,** Dispersing
Agent, Formulation Aid, Nutritive Sweetener, Tableting
Aid
Fumaric Acid - Acid, Acidifier, **Flavoring Agent**
Furfural - **Extraction Solvent**, **Flavoring Agent**

-G-
gamma-Butyrolcatone - **Flavoring Agent**
gamma-Heptalactone - **Flavoring Agent**
gamma-Nonalactone - **Flavoring Agent**
gamma-Octalactone - **Flavoring Agent**
gamma-Terpinene - **Flavoring Agent**
gamma-Undecalactone - **Flavoring Agent**
gamma-Valerolactone - **Flavoring Agent**
Garlic Oil - **Flavoring Agent**
Gellan Gum - **Gelling Agent**, Stabilizer, Suspending
Agent, Thickener
Geraniol - **Flavoring Agent**
Geranium Oil, Algerian Type - **Flavoring Agent**
Gerannyl Benzoate - **Flavoring Agent**
Geranyl Acetate - **Flavoring Agent**
Geranyl Acetoacetate - **Flavoring Agent**
Geranyl Butyrate - **Flavoring Agent**
Geranyl Formate - **Flavoring Agent**

Geranyl Phenylacetate - **Flavoring Agent**
Geranyl Propionate - **Flavoring Agent**
Gibberellic Acid - Enzyme Activator
Ginger Oil - **Flavoring Agent**
Glucono Delta-Lactone - **Acid**, Acidifier, Leavening Agent, Sequestrant
Glucono delta-Lactone - **Acid**, Acidifier, Leavening Agent
Glucose Isomerase (Actinoplanes Missouriensis) - **Enzyme**
Glucose Isomerase (Bacillus Coagulans) - **Enzyme**
Glucose Isomerase (Streptomyces Olivaceous) - **Enzyme**
Glucose Isomerase (Streptomyces Olivochromogenes) - **Enzyme**
Glucose Isomerase (Streptomyces Rubiginosus) - **Enzyme**
Glucose Isomerase (Streptomyces Violaceoniger) - **Enzyme**
Glucose Oxidase (Aspergillus Niger Var.) - **Enzyme**
Glycerin - **Binder**, Bodying Agent, Bulking Agent, Filler, Humectant, Moisture-Retaining Agent, Plasticizer, Solubilizer, Solvent, Vehicle
Glycerol - Bodying Agent, Bulking Agent, Carrier Solvent, Humectant, Moisture-Retaining Agent
Glycerol Diacetate - **Carrier Solvent**
Glycerol Ester of Partially Dimerized Rosin - Chewing Gum Base Component
Glycerol Ester of Partially Hydrogenated Wood Rosin - Chewing Gum Base Component
Glycerol Ester of Polymerized Rosin - Chewing Gum Base Component
Glycerol Ester of Tall Oil Rosin - Chewing Gum Base Component
Glycerol Ester of Wood Rosin - Chewing Gum Base Component, Stabilizer, Suspending Agent
Glycine - **Dietary Supplement**, Nutrient
Grape Skin Extract - **Color**

Grapefruit Oil, Coldpressed - **Flavoring Agent**
Green S - **Color**
Guaiac Resin - Antioxidant
Guar Gum - **Emulsifier**, Foaming Agent, Gelling Agent, Stabilizer, Suspending Agent, Thickener, Whipping Agent
Gum Arabic - **Gelling Agent**, Stabilizer, Suspending Agent, Thickener
Gum Ghatti - **Gelling Agent**, Stabilizer, Suspending Agent, Thickener
Gum Guaiac - Antioxidant, **Preservative**

-H-
Hemicellulase (Aspergillus Niger, Var.) - Enzyme
Heptanal - **Flavoring Agent**
Heptane - **Extraction Solvent**
Heptyl Alcohol - **Flavoring Agent**
Heptylparaben - Antimicrobial Agent, Preservative
Hexabe - **Extraction Solvent**
Hexanal - **Flavoring Agent**
Hexanoic Aacid - **Flavoring Agent**
Hexxyl-2-Buutenoate **Flavoring Agent**
Hexyl 2-Methylbutyrate - **Flavoring Agent**
Hexyl Alcohol, Natural - **Flavoring Agent**
Hexyl Isovalerate - **Flavoring Agent**
Hops Oil - **Flavoring Agent**
Hydrochloric Acid - **Acid,** Acidifier
Hydrogen Peroxide - **Bleaching Agent,** Oxidizing Agent, Starch-Modifying Agent
Hydroxycitronellal - **Flavoring Agent**
Hydroxycitronellal Dimethyl Acetal - **Flavoring Agent**
Hydroxycitronellol - **Flavoring Agent**
Hydroxylated Lecithin - Cloud Producing Agent, **Emulsifier**, Foaming Agent, Whipping Agent

Hydroxypropyl Cellulose - Coating Agent, **Emulsifier**, Film Former, Foaming Agent, Gelling Agent, Glaze, Polish, Stabilizer, Surface-Finishing Agent, Suspending Agent, Thickener, Whipping Agent

Hydroxypropyl Distarch Phosphate - **Binder**, Filler, Gelling Agent, Plasticizer, Stabilizer, Suspending Agent, Thickener

Hydroxypropyl Methyl Cellulose - **Emulsifier**, Foaming Agent, Gelling Agent, Thickener, Whipping Agent

Hydroxypropyl Methylcellulose - **Emulsifier**, Foaming Agent, Gelling Agent, Stabilizer, Suspending Agent, Thickener, Whipping Agent

Hydroxypropyl Starch - Binder, **Emulsifier**, Filler, Foaming Agent, Gelling Agent, Plasticizer, Thickener, Whipping Agent

Hydroxypropylmethyl Cellulose - Stabilizer, Suspending Agent

-I-

Indigotine - Color

Indole - **Flavoring Agent**

Inositol - **Dietary Supplement**, Nutrient

Insoluble Polyvinylpyrrolidone - Colloidal Stabilizer, Color Stabilizer

Iron Oxide Red - Color

Iron Oxide Yellow - Color

Iron Oxides - Color

Iron, Carbonyl - **Dietary Supplement**, Nutrient

Iron, Electrolytic - **Dietary Supplement**, Nutrient

Iron, Reduced - **Dietary Supplement**, Nutrient

Iso-alpha-Methyl Ionone - **Flavoring Agent**

Isoamyl Acetate - **Flavoring Agent**

Isoamyl Butyrate - **Flavoring Agent**

Isoamyl Formate - **Flavoring Agent**

Isoamyl Gallate - Antioxidant

Isoamyl Hexanoate - **Flavoring Agent**

Isoamyl Isovalerate - **Flavoring Agent**
Isoamyl Salicylate - **Flavoring Agent**
Isobornyl Acetate - **Flavoring Agent**
Isobutanol - **Extraction Solvent**
Isobutyl Acetate - **Flavoring Agent**
Isobutyl Alcohol - **Flavoring Agent**
Isobutyl Butyrate - **Flavoring Agent**
Isobutyl Cinnamate - **Flavoring Agent**
Isobutyl Phenylacetate - **Flavoring Agent**
Isobutyl Salicylate - **Flavoring Agent**
Isobutyl-2-Butenoate - **Flavoring Agent**
Isobutylene-Isoprene Copolymer - Chewing Gum Base Component
Isobutyraldehyde - **Flavoring Agent**
Isobutyric Acid - **Flavoring Agent**
Isoeugenol - **Flavoring Agent**
Isoeugenyl Acetate - **Flavoring Agent**
Isomalt - **Sweetening Agent**
Isopropyl Acetate - **Extraction Solvent**, **Flavoring Agent**
Isopropyl Alcohol - Solubilizer, Solvent, Vehicle
Isopropyl Citrate Mixture - Antioxidant, Sequestrant
Isopropyl Myristate - Carrier Solvent
Isopulegol - **Flavoring Agent**
Isoquinoline - **Flavoring Agent**
Isovaleric Acid - **Flavoring Agent**

-J-
Juniper Berry Oil - **Flavoring Agent**

-K-
Kaolin - Anticaking Agent, Drying Agent
Karaya Gum - **Emulsifier**, Foaming Agent, Gelling Agent, Stabilizer, Suspending Agent, Thickener, Whipping Agent

Kelp - **Dietary Supplement**, Nutrient

-L-
L(+)-Tartaric Acid - Acid, Acidifier, Antioxidant Synergist, Sequestrant
L-Alanine - **Dietary Supplement**, Nutrient
L-Arginine - **Dietary Supplement**, Nutrient
L-Arginine Monohydrochloride - **Dietary Supplement**, Nutrient
L-Asparagine - **Dietary Supplement**, Nutrient
L-Aspartic Acid - **Dietary Supplement**, Nutrient
L-Carvone - **Flavoring Agent**
L-Cysteine Monohydrochloride - **Dietary Supplement**, Nutrient
L-Cystine - **Dietary Supplement**, Nutrient
L-Glutamic Acid - **Dietary Supplement**, Flavor Enhancer, Intensifier, Nutrient, Salt Substitute
L-Glutamic Acid Hydrochloride - **Dietary Supplement**, **Flavoring Agent**, Nutrient, Salt Substitute
L-Glutamine - **Dietary Supplement**, Nutrient
L-Histidine - **Dietary Supplement**, Nutrient
L-Histidine Monohydrochloride - **Dietary Supplement**, Nutrient
L-Isoleucine - **Dietary Supplement**, Nutrient
L-Leucine - **Dietary Supplement**, Nutrient
L-Limonene - **Flavoring Agent**
L-Lysine Monohydrochloride - **Dietary Supplement**, Nutrient
L-Menthol - **Flavoring Agent**
L-Menthone - **Flavoring Agent**
L-Menthyl Acetate - **Flavoring Agent**
L-Methionine - **Dietary Supplement**, Nutrient
L-Phenylalanine - **Dietary Supplement**, Nutrient
L-Proline - **Dietary Supplement**, Nutrient
L-Serine - **Dietary Supplement**, Nutrient
L-Threonine - **Dietary Supplement**, Nutrient

L-Tryptophan - **Dietary Supplement**, Nutrient
L-Tyrosine - **Dietary Supplement**, Nutrient
L-Valine - **Dietary Supplement**, Nutrient
Labdanum Oil - **Flavoring Agent**
Lactated Mono-Diglycerides - **Emulsifier**, Foaming
Agent, Stabilizer, Suspending Agent, Whipping Agent
Lactic Acid - Acid, Acidifier
Lactic and Fatty Acid Esters of Glycerol - **Emulsifier**,
Foaming Agent, Whipping Agent
Lactitol - **Sweetening Agent**, Texture-Modifying Agent,
Texturizer
Lactylated Fatty Acid Esters of Glycerol and Propylene
Glycol - Binder, **Emulsifier**, Filler, Foaming Agent,
Plasticizer, Stabilizer, Surface-Active Agent, Suspending
Agent, Wetting Agent, Whipping Agent
Lactylic Esters of Fatty Acids - **Emulsifier**, Foaming
Agent, Surface-Active Agent, Wetting Agent, Whipping
Agent
Lanolin, Anyhydrous - Chewing Gum Base Component
Laurel Leaf Oil - **Flavoring Agent**
Lauric Acid - Component in the Manufacture of Other
Food-Grade, Additives, Defoaming Agent, **Flavoring
Agent**
Lecithin - Antioxidant, **Emulsifier**, Foaming Agent,
Whipping Agent
Lecithin, Partially Hydrolyzed Antioxidant, **Emulsifier**,
Foaming Agent, Whipping Agent
Lemon Oil, Coldpressed - **Flavoring Agent**
Lemon Oil, Desert Type, Coldpressed - **Flavoring Agent**
Lemon Oil, Distilled - **Flavoring Agent**
Lemongrass Oil - **Flavoring Agent**
Light Petroleum - **Extraction Solvent**
Lime Oil, Coldpressed - **Flavoring Agent**
Lime Oil, Distilled - **Flavoring Agent**
Limestone, Ground - Chewing Gum Base Component
Linaloe Wood Oil - **Flavoring Agent**

Linalool - **Flavoring Agent**
Linalyl Acetate - **Flavoring Agent**
Linalyl Acetate, Synthetic - **Flavoring Agent**
Linalyl Benzoate - **Flavoring Agent**
Linalyl Formate - **Flavoring Agent**
Linalyl Isobutyrate - **Flavoring Agent**
Linalyl Propionate - **Flavoring Agent**
Lipase - Enzyme
Lipase (Aspergillus Niger Var.) - Enzyme
Lipase (Aspergillus Oryzae Var.) - Enzyme
Lithol Rubine BK - Color
Locust (Carob) Bean Gum - **Emulsifier**, Foaming Agent, Gelling Agent, Stabilizer, Suspending Agent, Thickener, Whipping Agent
Lovage Oil - **Flavoring Agent**

-M-
Mace Oil - **Flavoring Agent**
Magnesium Carbonate - Alkali, Antibleaching Agent, Anticaking Agent, Carrier, Disintegrating Agent, Dispersing Agent, Drying Agent, Formulation Aid, Tableting Aid
Magnesium Chloride - Color Retention Agent, **Firming Agent**
Magnesium Di-L-Glutamate - Flavor Enhancer, Intensifier, Salt Substitute
Magnesium DL-Lactate - Buffer, **Dietary Supplement**, Dough Conditioner, Neutralizing Agent
Magnesium Gluconate - Buffer, **Firming Agent**, Neutralizing Agent, Yeast Food
Magnesium Hydrogen Carbonate - Carrier, Color Retention Agent, Disintegrating Agent, Dispersing Agent, Formulation Aid, Tableting Aid
Magnesium Hydrogen Phosphate - **Dietary Supplement**, Nutrient

Magnesium Hydroxide - Alkali, Anticaking Agent, Color Adjunct, Drying Agent

Magnesium Hydroxide Carbonate - Alkali, Anticaking Agent, Drying Agent

Magnesium L-Lactate - Buffer, **Dietary Supplement**, Dough Conditioner, Neutralizing Agent

Magnesium Oxide - Alkali, Anticaking Agent, Buffer, Drying Agent, Neutralizing Agent

Magnesium Phosphate, Dibasic - **Dietary Supplement**, Nutrient

Magnesium Phosphate, Tribasic - **Dietary Supplement**, Nutrient

Magnesium Silicate - **Filter Aid**

Magnesium Silicate (Synthetic) - Anticaking Agent, Drying Agent

Magnesium Stearate - Anticaking Agent, Binder, Drying Agent, **Emulsifier**, Filler, Foaming Agent, Plasticizer, Whipping Agent

Magnesium Sulfate - **Dietary Supplement**, Nutrient

Malic Acid - Acid, Acidifier, **Flavoring Agent**

Malt - **Enzyme**

Malt Carbohydrases - **Enzyme**

Maltilol - **Humectant**, Moisture-Retaining Agent

Maltilol Syrup - **Sweetening Agent**

Maltitol - **Sweetening Agent**

Maltol - **Flavoring Agent**

Mandarin Oil, Coldpressed - **Flavoring Agent**

Manganese Chloride - **Dietary Supplement**, Nutrient

Manganese Gluconate - **Dietary Supplement**, Nutrient

Manganese Glycerophosphate - **Dietary Supplement**, Nutrient

Manganese Hypophosphite - **Dietary Supplement**, Nutrient

Manganese Sulfate - **Dietary Supplement**, Nutrient

Mannitol - **Dietary Supplement**, Humectant, Moisture-Retaining Agent, Nutrient, **Sweetening Agent**, Texture-Modifying Agent, Texturizer

Marjoram Oil, Spanish Type - **Flavoring Agent**

Marjoram Oil, Sweet - **Flavoring Agent**

Masticatory Substances, Natural - Chewing Gum Base Component

Mentha Arvensis Oil, Partially Dementholized - **Flavoring Agent**

Menthol - **Flavoring Agent**

Methanol - **Extraction Solvent**

Methycellulose - Bodying Agent, Bulking Agent

Methyl 2-Methylbutyrate - **Flavoring Agent**

Methyl 2-Octynoate - **Flavoring Agent**

Methyl Alcohol - Solubilizer, Solvent, Vehicle

Methyl Anthranilate - **Flavoring Agent**

Methyl Benzoate - **Flavoring Agent**

Methyl beta-Naphthyl Ketone - **Flavoring Agent**

Methyl Cellulose - **Emulsifier**, Foaming Agent, Gelling Agent, Stabilizer, Suspending Agent, Thickener, Whipping Agent

Methyl Cinnamate - **Flavoring Agent**

Methyl Cyclopentenoione - **Flavoring Agent**

Methyl Ester of Rosin, Partially Hydrogenated - Chewing Gum Base Component

Methyl Ethyl Cellulose - Gelling Agent, Stabilizer,

Methyl Eugenol - **Flavoring Agent**

Methyl Isoeugenol - **Flavoring Agent**

Methyl N-Methyl Anthranilate - **Flavoring Agent**

Methyl Phenylacetate - **Flavoring Agent**

Methyl Phenylcarbinyl Acetate - **Flavoring Agent**

Methylbenzyl Acetate - **Flavoring Agent**

Methylcellulose - Binder, Coating Agent, **Emulsifier**, Filler, Film Former, Foaming Agent, Gelling Agent, Glaze, Plasticizer, Polish, Stabilizer, Surface-Finishing Agent, Suspending Agent, Thickener, Whipping Agent

Methylene Chloride - Solubilizer, Solvent, Vehicle

Methylparaben - Antimicrobial Agent, Preservative

Microcrystalline Cellulose - Anticaking Agent, Carrier, Disintegrating Agent, Dispersing Agent, Drying Agent, **Emulsifier**, Foaming Agent, Formulation Aid, Tableting Aid, Whipping Agent

Mineral Oil - Release Agent, Sealing Agent

Mineral Oil, White - Antisticking Agent, Binder, Coating Agent, Defoaming Agent, Filler, Film Former, Glaze, Lubricant, Plasticizer, Polish, Release Agent, Surface-Finishing Agent

Mixed Carbohydrase and Protease (Bacillus Subtilis) - Enzyme

Modified Starch - Gelling Agent, Thickener

Modified Starches - Binder, Filler, Plasticizer, Stabilizer, Suspending Agent

Mono- and Diglycerides - **Emulsifier**, Foaming Agent, Stabilizer, Suspending Agent, Whipping Agent

Monoammonium L-Glutamate - Flavor Enhancer, Intensifier, Salt Substitute

Monoglyceride Citrate - Antioxidant Solubilizer, Flavor Solubilizer

Monopotassium L-Glutamate - Flavor Enhancer, Intensifier, Salt Substitute

Monosodium L-Glutamate - Flavor Enhancer, Intensifier

Monostarch Phosphate - Binder, Filler, Gelling Agent, Plasticizer, Stabilizer, Suspending Agent, Thickener

Myrcene - **Flavoring Agent**
Myristic Acid - Component in the Manufacture of Other Food-Grade, Additives, Defoaming Agent, **Flavoring Agent**
Myrrh Oil - **Flavoring Agent**

-N-
N-Acetyl-L-Methionine - **Dietary Supplement**, Nutrient
Nerol - **Flavoring Agent**
Nerolidol - **Flavoring Agent**
Niacin - **Dietary Supplement**, Nutrient
Niacinamide - **Dietary Supplement**, Nutrient
Niacinamide Ascorbate - **Dietary Supplement**, Nutrient
Nisin - Preservative
Nitrogen - Freezant, Packing Gas
Nitrous Oxide - Propellant
Nonanal - **Flavoring Agent**
Nonyl Acetate - **Flavoring Agent**
Nonyl Alcohol - **Flavoring Agent**
Nordihydroguaiaretic Acid - Antioxidant
Nutmeg Oil - **Flavoring Agent**

-O-
O-Phenylphenol - Preservative
Octanal - **Flavoring Agent**
Octanoic Acid - Component in the Manufacture of Other Food-Grade, Additives, Defoaming Agent, **Flavoring Agent**
Octyl Acetate - **Flavoring Agent**
Octyl Formate - **Flavoring Agent**
Octyl Gallate - Antioxidant
Oleic Acid - Antisticking Agent, Binder, Component in the Manufacture of Other Food-Grade, Additives, Defoaming Agent, Filler, Lubricant, Plasticizer, Release Agent
Oleoresin Black Pepper - **Flavoring Agent**
Oleoresin Capsicum - **Flavoring Agent**

Oleoresin Celery - **Flavoring Agent**
Oleoresin Ginger - **Flavoring Agent**
Oleoresin Paprika - **Flavoring Agent**
Oleoresin Turmeric - **Flavoring Agent**
Olibanum Oil - **Flavoring Agent**
Onion Oil - **Flavoring Agent**
Orange GGN - Color
Orange Oil, Bitter, Coldpressed - **Flavoring Agent**
Orange Oil, Coldpressed - **Flavoring Agent**
Orange Oil, Distilled Origanum Oil, Spanish Type -
Flavoring Agent
Orris Root Oil - **Flavoring Agent**
Oxidized Starch - Binder, Filler, Gelling Agent,
Plasticizer, Thickener
Oxidized Starch Polyglycerol Esters of Interesterified
Ricinoleic Acid - **Emulsifier**, Foaming Agent, Whipping
Agent
Oxystearin - Antifoaming Agent, Defoaming Agent,
Sequestrant

-P-
P-Methoxybenzaldehyde - **Flavoring Agent**
P-Methyl Anisole - **Flavoring Agent**
P-Propyl Anisole - **Flavoring Agent**
P-Propylanisole - **Flavoring Agent**
P-Tolyl Isobutyrate - **Flavoring Agent**
Palmarosa Oil - **Flavoring Agent**
Palmitic Acid - Component in the Manufacture of Other
Food-Grade, Additives, Defoaming Agent
Papain - Enzyme
Paprika Oleoresins - Color, **Flavoring Agent**
Paraffin Wax - Chewing Gum Base Component,
Defoaming Agent
Paraffin, Synthetic - Chewing Gum Base Component
Parsley Herb Oil - **Flavoring Agent**
Parsley Seed Oil - **Flavoring Agent**

Patent Blue V - Color
Pectin - **Emulsifier**, Foaming Agent, Gelling Agent, Stabilizer, Suspending Agent, Thickener, Whipping Agent
Pectinases (Aspergillus Niger, Var.) - Enzyme
Pennyroyal Oil - **Flavoring Agent**
Pentaerythritol Ester of Wood Rosin - Chewing Gum Base Component
Pentapotassium Triphosphate - Texture-Modifying Agent, Texturizer
Pentasodium Triphosphate - Texture-Modifying Agent, Texturizer
Peppermint Oil - **Flavoring Agent**
Pepsin - Enzyme
Perlite - Filter Aid
Petitgrain Oil, Paraguay Type - **Flavoring Agent**
Petrolatum - Antisticking Agent, Coating Agent, Defoaming Agent, Film Former, Glaze, Lubricant, Polish, Release Agent, Surface-Finishing Agent
Petroleum Jelly - Antifoaming Agent, Antisticking Agent, Lubricant, Release Agent, Sealing Agent
Petroleum Wax - Chewing Gum Base Component, Coating Agent, Defoaming Agent, Film Former, Glaze, Polish, Surface-Finishing Agent
Petroleum Wax, Synthetic Chewing Gum Base Component, Coating Agent, Defoaming Agent, Film Former, Glaze, Polish, Surface-Finishing Agent
Phenethyl Acetate - **Flavoring Agent**
Phenethyl Alcohol - **Flavoring Agent**
Phenethyl Isobutyrate - **Flavoring Agent**
Phenethyl Isovalerate - **Flavoring Agent**
Phenylacetaldehyde - **Flavoring Agent**
Phenylacetaldehyde Dimethyl Acetal **Flavoring Agent**
Phenylacetic Acid **Flavoring Agent**
Phosphated Distarch Phosphate - Binder, Filler, Gelling Agent, Plasticizer, Stabilizer, Suspending Agent, Thickener

hosphoric Acid - Acid, Acidifier, Antioxidant Synergist, Sequestrant
Pimaricin - Fungicidal Preservative
Pimenta Leaf Oil F- lavoring Agent
Pimenta Oil - **Flavoring Agent**
Pine Needle Oil, Dwarf - **Flavoring Agent**
Pine Needle Oil, Scotch Type - **Flavoring Agent**
Piperonal - **Flavoring Agent**
Poloxamer 331 - Flavoring Adjunct or Adjuvant, Solubilizer, Solvent, Stabilizer, Suspending Agent, Vehicle
Poloxamer 407 - Flavoring Adjunct or Adjuvant, Solubilizer, Solvent, Stabilizer, Suspending Agent, Vehicle
Polydextroses - Bodying Agent, Bulking Agent, Carrier, Disintegrating Agent, Dispersing Agent, Formulation Aid, Gelling Agent, Stabilizer, Suspending Agent, Tableting Aid, Texture-Modifying Agent, Texturizer, Thickener
Polydimethylsiloxane - Anticaking Agent, Antifoaming Agent, Drying Agent
Polyethylene - Chewing Gum Base Component
Polyethylene Glycols - Antisticking Agent, Binder, Carrier, Carrier Solvent, Coating Agent, Disintegrating Agent, Dispersing Agent, Filler, Film Former, Flavoring Adjunct or Adjuvant, Formulation Aid, Glaze, Lubricant, Plasticizer, Polish, Release Agent, Surface-Finishing Agent, Tableting Aid
Polyglycerol Esters of Fatty Acids - **Emulsifier**, Foaming Agent, Whipping Agent
Polyisobutylene - Chewing Gum Base Component
Polyoxyethylene (20) Sorbitan Monolaurate - Carrier, Disintegrating Agent, Dispersing Agent, **Emulsifier**, Foaming Agent, Formulation Aid, Tableting Aid, Whipping Agent

Polyoxyethylene (20) Sorbitan Monooleate - Carrier, Disintegrating Agent, Dispersing Agent, **Emulsifier**, Foaming Agent, Formulation Aid, Tableting Aid, Whipping Agent

Polyoxyethylene (20) Sorbitan Monopalmitate - Carrier, Disintegrating Agent, Dispersing Agent, **Emulsifier**, Foaming Agent, Formulation Aid, Tableting Aid, Whipping Agent

Polyoxyethylene (20) Sorbitan Monostearate- Carrier, Disintegrating Agent, Dispersing Agent, **Emulsifier**, Foaming Agent, Formulation Aid, Tableting Aid, Whipping Agent

Polyoxyethylene (20) Sorbitan Tristearate - Carrier, Disintegrating Agent, Dispersing Agent, **Emulsifier**, Foaming Agent, Formulation Aid, Tableting Aid, Whipping Agent

Polyoxyethylene (40) Stearate - **Emulsifier**, Foaming Agent, Whipping Agent

Polyoxyethylene (8) Stearate - **Emulsifier**, Foaming Agent, Whipping Agent

Polypropylene Glycol - Defoaming Agent

-Q-

Quillaia Extracts - **Emulsifier**, Foaming Agent, Whipping Agent

Quinine Hydrochloride - **Flavoring Agent**

Quinine Sulfate - **Flavoring Agent**

Quinoline - Yellow Color

-R-

Red 2G - Color

Rennet - Enzyme

Rennet (Bacillus Cereus) - Enzyme

Rennet (Endothis Parasitica) - Enzyme

Rennet (Mucor Species) - Enzyme

Rennet, Bovine - Enzyme
Rhodinol - **Flavoring Agent**
Rhodinyl Acetate - **Flavoring Agent**
Rhodinyl Formate - **Flavoring Agent**
Riboflain - Color
Riboflavin - **Dietary Supplement**, Nutrient
Rice Bran Wax - Chewing Gum Base Component, Coating Agent, Film Former, Glaze, Polish, Surface-Finishing Agent
ose Oil - **Flavoring Agent**
Rosemary Oil - **Flavoring Agent**
Rue Oil - **Flavoring Agent**

-S-
Saccharin - Nonnutritive Sweetener, Sugar Substitute, **Sweetening Agent**
Saffron - Color
Sage Oil, Dalmatian Type - **Flavoring Agent**
Sage Oil, Spanish Type - **Flavoring Agent**
Salts of Fatty Acids - Anticaking Agent, Drying Agent, **Emulsifier**, Foaming Agent, Whipping Agent
Sandalwood Oil, East Indian Type - **Flavoring Agent**
Santalol - **Flavoring Agent**
Santalyl Acetate - **Flavoring Agent**
Savory Oil (Summer Variety) - **Flavoring Agent**
Shellac, Bleached - Coating Agent, Film Former, Glaze, Polish, Surface-Finishing Agent
Shellac, Bleached, Wax Free - Coating Agent, Film Former, Glaze, Polish, Surface-Finishing Agent
Silicon Dioxide - Anticaking Agent, Carrier, Defoaming Agent, Disintegrating Agent, Dispersing Agent, Drying Agent, Formulation Aid, Tableting Aid
Silicon Dioxide Amorphous - Anticaking Agent, Drying Agent
Smoke Flavorings - Color, **Flavoring Agent**

Sodiium Stearoyl Lactylate - Stabilizer, Suspending Agent
Sodium Acetate - Buffer, Neutralizing Agent
Sodium Acetate, Anhydrous - Buffer, Neutralizing Agent
Sodium Acid Pyrophosphate - Buffer, Leavening Agent, Neutralizing Agent, Sequestrant
Sodium Adipate - Buffer, Neutralizing Agent
Sodium Alginate - **Emulsifier**, Foaming Agent, Gelling Agent, Stabilizer, Suspending Agent, Thickener, Whipping Agent
Sodium Aluminosilicate - Anticaking Agent, Drying Agent
Sodium Aluminum Phosphate, Acidic - Leavening Agent
Sodium Aluminum Phosphate, Basic - **Emulsifier**, Foaming Agent, Whipping Agent
Sodium Ascorbate - Antioxidant, **Dietary Supplement**, Nutrient
Sodium Benzoate - Antimicrobial Agent, Preservative
Sodium Bicarbonate - Alkali, Leavening Agent
Sodium Bisulfate - Acid, Acidifier
Sodium Bisulfite - Preservative
Sodium Carbonate - Alkali
Sodium Carboxymethylcellulose - Gelling Agent, Stabilizer, Suspending Agent, Thickener
Sodium Caseinate - **Emulsifier**, Foaming Agent, Stabilizer, Suspending Agent, Whipping Agent
Sodium Chloride - **Dietary Supplement**, Dough Conditioner, Flavor Enhancer, Intensifier, **Flavoring Agent**, Nutrient
Sodium Citrate - Buffer, Neutralizing Agent, Sequestrant
Sodium Cyclamate - **Sweetening Agent**
Sodium Dehydroacetate - Preservative
Sodium Diacetate - Antimold Agent, Antirope Agent, Preservative, Sequestrant
Sodium Dihydrogen Citrate - Buffer, Neutralizing Agent, Sequestrant

Sodium Dihydrogen Phosphate - Buffer, Neutralizing
Agent, Sequestrant
Sodium DL-Malate - Buffer, Neutralizing Agent,
Seasoning
Agent
Sodium Erythorbate - Antioxidant, Preservative
Sodium Ferric Pyrophosphate - **Dietary Supplement**,
Nutrient
Sodium Ferrocyanide - Anticaking Agent, Drying Agent
Sodium Fumarate - Acid, Acidifier, Buffer, Neutralizing
Agent, Seasoning Agent
Sodium Gluconate - **Dietary Supplement**, Nutrient,
Sequestrant, Yeast Food
Sodium Hydrogen Carbonate - Alkali, Buffer, Leavening
Agent, Neutralizing Agent
Sodium Hydrogen DL-Malate - Buffer, Humectant,
Moisture-Retaining Agent, Neutralizing Agent
Sodium Hydrogen Sulfite - Antimicrobial Agent,
Preservative
Sodium Hydroxide - Alkali
Sodium Hydroxide Solution - Alkali
Sodium Hypophosphite - Antioxidant, Preservative
Sodium L(+)-Tartrate - Sequestrant, Stabilizer,
Suspending Agent
Sodium Lactate (Solution) - Antioxidant Synergist,
Bodying Agent, Bulking Agent, Humectant, Moisture-
Retaining Agent
Sodium Lauryl Sulfate - Surface-Active Agent, Wetting
Agent
Sodium Metabisulfite - Antimicrobial Agent, Antioxidant,
Bleaching Agent, Oxidizing Agent, Preservative
Sodium Metaphosphate, Insoluble - **Emulsifier**, Foaming
Agent, Sequestrant, Texture-Modifying Agent,
Texturizer, Whipping Agent

Sodium Nitrate - Antimicrobial Agent, Color Fixative, Preservative

Sodium Nitrite - Antimicrobial Agent, Color Fixative, Preservative

Sodium O-Phenylphenol - Preservative

Sodium Phosphate, Dibasic - Buffer, **Dietary Supplement**, **Emulsifier**, Foaming Agent, Neutralizing Agent, Nutrient, Texture-Modifying Agent, Texturizer, Whipping Agent

Sodium Phosphate, Monobasic - Buffer, **Dietary Supplement**, **Emulsifier**, Foaming Agent, Neutralizing Agent, Nutrient, Whipping Agent

Sodium Phosphate, Tribasic - Buffer, **Dietary Supplement**, **Emulsifier**, Foaming Agent, Neutralizing Agent, Nutrient, Whipping Agent

Sodium Polyphosphates, Glassy - **Emulsifier**, Foaming Agent, Sequestrant, Texture-Modifying Agent, Texturizer, Whipping Agent

Sodium Potassium Tartrate - , Neutralizing Agent, Sequestrant

Sodium Propionate - Antimicrobial Agent, Antimold Agent, Antirope Agent, Preservative

Sodium Pyrophosphate - Buffer, **Dietary Supplement**, **Emulsifier**, Foaming Agent, Neutralizing Agent, Nutrient, Whipping Agent

Sodium Saccharin - Nonnutritive Sweetener, Sugar Substitute, **Sweetening Agent**

Sodium Sesquicarbonate - Alkali, Buffer, Neutralizing Agent

Sodium Stearoyl Lactylate Dough Conditioner, **Emulsifier**, Foaming Agent, Whipping Agent

Sodium Stearyl Fumarate - Dough Conditioner

Sodium Sulfate - Component in the Manufacture of Other Food-Grade Additives

-T-

Tagetes Extract - Color

Talc - Anticaking Agent, Antisticking Agent, Coating Agent,
Drying Agent, Dusting Powder, Film Former, Filter Aid, Glaze, Lubricant, Polish, Release Agent, Surface-Finishing Agent, Texture-Modifying Agent, Texturizer

Tangerine Oil, Coldpressed - **Flavoring Agent**

Tannic Acid - Clarifying Agent

Tara Gum - Gelling Agent, Stabilizer, Suspending Agent, Thickener

Tarragon Oil - **Flavoring Agent**

Tartaric Acid - Acid, Acidifier, Sequestrant

Tartrazine - Color

TBHQ - Antioxidant

Terpene Resine, Natural - Chewing Gum Base Component

Terpene Resine, Synthetic - Chewing Gum Base Component

Terpineol - **Flavoring Agent**

Terpinyl Acetate - **Flavoring Agent**

Terpinyl Propionate - **Flavoring Agent**

Tertiary Butylhydroquinone - Antioxidant

Tetrahydrolinalool - **Flavoring Agent**

Tetrapotassium Pyrophosphate - Buffer, **Emulsifier**, Foaming Agent, Neutralizing Agent, Whipping Agent

Tetrasodium Pyrophosphate - Anticaking Agent, Buffer, Drying Agent, **Emulsifier**, Foaming Agent, Neutralizing Agent, Sequestrant, Whipping Agent

Thaumatin - Flavor Enhancer, Intensifier, **Sweetening Agent**

Thiamin Hydrochloride - **Dietary Supplement**, Nutrient

Thiamin Mononitrate - **Dietary Supplement**, Nutrient

Thiodipropionic Acid - Antioxidant

Thyme Oil - **Flavoring Agent**
Titanium Dioxide - Color
Tocopherols, Mixed - Antioxidant, **Dietary Supplement**, Nutrient
Toluene - **Extraction Solvent**
Tragacanth - **Emulsifier**, Foaming Agent, Gelling Agent, Stabilizer, Suspending Agent, Thickener, Whipping Agent
Tragacanth Gum - **Emulsifier**, Foaming Agent, Stabilizer, Suspending Agent, Whipping Agent
Trans,Cis-2,6-Nonadienal - **Flavoring Agent**
Trans,Cis-2,6-Nonadienol - **Flavoring Agent**
Trans,Trans-2,4-Decadienal - **Flavoring Agent**
Trans,Trans-2,4-Heptadienal - **Flavoring Agent**
Trans,Trans-2,4-Nonadienal - **Flavoring Agent**
Trans-2-Decen-1-Al - **Flavoring Agent**
Trans-2-Dodecen-1-Al - **Flavoring Agent**
Trans-2-Hexen-1-Al - **Flavoring Agent**
Trans-2-Hexen-1-Ol - **Flavoring Agent**
Trans-2-Nonen-1-Ol - **Flavoring Agent**
Trans-2-Nonenal - **Flavoring Agent**
Trans-2-Octen-1-Al - **Flavoring Agent**
Trans-Anethole - **Flavoring Agent**
Triacetin - Carrier Solvent, Humectant, Moisture-Retaining Agent, Solubilizer, Solvent, Vehicle
Triammonium Citrate - Buffer, Neutralizing Agent.
Tributyrin - **Flavoring Agent**
Tricalcium Phosphate - Anticaking Agent, Buffer, Drying Agent, Neutralizing Agent
Trichloroethylene - **Extraction Solvent**, Solubilizer, Solvent, Vehicle
Trichlorogalactosucrose - **Sweetening Agent**
Triethyl Citrate - Carrier Solvent, Sequestrant
Trimagnesium Phosphate - Anticaking Agent, Drying Agent
Tripotassium Citrate - Buffer, Neutralizing Agent, Sequestrant, Stabilizer, Suspending Agent

Tripotassium Phosphate - Buffer, Emulsion Stabilizer, Neutralizing Agent, Sequestrant

Trisodium Citrate - Buffer, **Emulsifier**, Foaming Agent, Neutralizing Agent, Sequestrant, Stabilizer, Suspending Agent, Whipping Agent

Trisodium Phosphate - Buffer, **Emulsifier**, Foaming Agent, Neutralizing Agent, Sequestrant, Stabilizer, Suspending Agent, Whipping Agent

Trypsin - Enzyme

Turmeric - Color

Turmeric Oleoresin - Color, **Flavoring Agent**

-U-

Undecanal - **Flavoring Agent**

Undecyl Alcohol - **Flavoring Agent**

-V-

Valeric Acid - **Flavoring Agent**

Vanillin - **Flavoring Agent**

Vitamin A - **Dietary Supplement**, Nutrient

Vitamin B12 - **Dietary Supplement**, Nutrient

Vitamin D2 - **Dietary Supplement**, Nutrient

Vitamin D3 - **Dietary Supplement**, Nutrient

-W-

Wintergreen Oil - **Flavoring Agent**

-X-

Xanthan Gum - Bodying Agent, Bulking Agent, **Emulsifier**, Foaming Agent, Gelling Agent, Stabilizer, Suspending Agent, Thickener, Whipping Agent

Xylitol - Humectant, Moisture-Retaining Agent, Nutritive Sweetener, **Sweetening Agent**

-Y-

- Z-
Zinc Gluconate - **Dietary Supplement**, Nutrient
Zinc Oxide - **Dietary Supplement**, Nutrient
Zinc Sulfate - **Dietary Supplement**, Nutrient

References

1. Shibamoto T, Bjeldanes LF. Introduction to Food Toxicology. 1993, Academic Press, San Diego, California

2. Watson DH, Ed. Natural Toxicants in Food. Progress and Prospects. Ellis Horwood Series in Food Science and Toxicology.

3. Liener IE. Implications of antinutritional components in soybean foods. Critical Reviews in Food Science and Nutrition 1994;34(1):31-67.

4. Concon JM. Food Science and Toxicology. Part A Principles and Concepts. 1988 Marcel Dekker, New York.

5. David Lary & Ralf Toumi,The atmospheric chemistry of HCN, CN and NCO,http:// www.atm.ch.cam.ac.uk /acmsu/newsletter11/ news8.html

6. Heaney Rk, Fenwick GR. Natural toxins and protective factors in Brassica species, including rapeseed. Natural Toxins 1995;3(4):233-237.

7. Seawright AA. Directly toxic effects of plants chemicals which may occur in human and animals foods. *Natural Toxins* 1995;3:227-232.

8. Data from Endometriosis Association Research Registry, partially published in Endometriosis Association Newsletter 10:2, 1989.

9. Hysterectomies in the United States, 1965-84. Vital and Health Statistics, U.S. Dept of Health and Human Services, Public Health Service, Centers for Disease Control, National Center for Health Statistics, Series 13, No. 92, 1987.

10. Older J. "Leeches and Laudanum: Grandmother and You: Historical Highlights." Endometriosis. (New York: Scribners, 1984)

11. Lamb K, Hoffmann RG, Nichols TR. "Family Trait Analysis: A Case-Control Study of 43 Women with Endometriosis and Their Best Friends." American Journal of Obstetrics and Gynecology 154: 3, 596-601, March 1986.

12. Nichols TR, Lamb K, Arkins JA. "The Association of Atopic Diseases with Endometriosis." Annals of Allergy 59:11, November 1987.

13. Lamb K, Nichols TR. "Endometriosis: A Comparison of Associated Disease Histories." American Journal of Preventive Medicine 2:6, 1986.

14. Ballweg ML. "A Heart Defect in Endometriosis: Another Clue to a Bigger Picture" Overcoming Endometriosis: Help from the Endometriosis Association. (New York: Congdon & Weed, Inc. 1987) pp. 228-231.

15. Fletcher N. "Mitral Valve Prolapse." Endometriosis Association Newsletter 13:2, 1992.

16. Ballweg ML. "Fibromyalgia/Endometriosis Link?..." Endometriosis Association Newsletter 12:3, 1991

17. Ballweg ML. "The Endometriosis- Candidiasis Link." Overcoming Endometriosis: New Help from the Endometriosis Association. (New York: Congdon & Weed, Inc., 1987), pp.198-219.

18. Grimes DA, Lebolt SA, Grimes KRT, and Wingo PA: "Two-fold risk of endometriosis in hospitalized patients with lupus." American Journal of Obstetrics and Gynecology 153: 179, 1985.

19. Brush MG, Department of Gynaecology, St. Thomas Hospital Medical School, London: "Increased Incidence of Thyroid Autoimmune Problems in Women with Endometriosis." Endometriosis: A Collection of Papers Written by GPs, Researchers, Specialists and Sufferers about Endometriosis. Compiled by the Coventry Branch of the Endometriosis Society, March 1987.

20. Fanton JW and Golden JG. "Radiation-induced endometriosis in Macaca mulatta." Radiation Research 126: 141-46, 1991.

21. Fanton JW, Hubbard GB, Wood DH. "Endometriosis: Clinical and pathological findings in 70 rhesus monkeys." American Journal of Veterinary Research 47: 1537-1541, 1986.

22. Campbell JS, Wong J, Tryphonas L, et al. "Is Simian Endometriosis an Effect of Immunotoxicity?" Presented at the Ontario Association of Pathologists Forty-Eighth Annual Meeting, October 1985, London, Ontario

23. Campbell J. "Is Reproductive Wastage and Failure Related to Environmental Pollution? - Considerations of human data and findings from a rhesus model." Symposium, Ottawa: "Toxicological Pathology - Quo Vadis?" September 1988.

24. Rier SE, Martin DC, Bowman RE, Dmowski WP, Becker JL. "Endometriosis in Rhesus Monkeys (Macaca mulatta) Following Chronic Exposure to 2,3,7,8-Tetrachlorodibenzo-p-dioxin." Fundamental and Applied Toxicology 21: 433-441, 1993

25. Rier SE, Spangelo BL, Martin DC, Bowman RE, Becker JL. "Tumor necrosis factor alpha and interleukin-6 production by peripheral blood mononuclear cells from rhesus monkeys with endometriosis." Journal of Immunology 150:49A, 1993

26. "Effects of estrogen, progesterone, and methoxychlor on surgically induced endometriosis in rats." Fundamental and Applied Toxicology 27:287-290, 1995

27. Cummings AM, Metcalf JL, and Birnbaum L. "Promotion of Endometriosis by 2,3,7,8-Tetrachlorodibenzo-p-dioxin in rats and mice: time-dose dependence and species comparison." Toxicology and Applied Pharmacology 138:131-139, 1996.

28. Johnson KL, Cummings AM, Birnbaum LS. "Promotion of endometriosis in mice by polychlorinated dibenzo-p-dioxins, dibenzofurans, and biphenyls." Environmental Health Perspectives 105(7):750-755, July 1997

29. Mayani A, Barel S, Soback S, et al. "Dioxin concentrations in women with endometriosis." Human Reproduction 12(3):373-375, 1997.

30. Cummings AM, Metcalf JL. "Induction of endometriosis in mice: a new model sensitive to estrogen." Reproductive Toxicology 9(3):233-238, 1995

31. Koninckx PR, Braet P, Kennedy SH, et al. "Dioxin pollution and endometriosis in Belgium." Human Reproduction 9(6):1001-1002, 1994

32. Rier SE, Martin DC, Bowman RE, et al. "Immunoresponsiveness in endometriosis: implications of estrogenic toxicants." Environmental Health Perspectives 103(supp. 7):151-156, October 1995.

33. Swain Wayland R. "Human health consequences of consumption of fish contaminated with organochlorine compounds." Aquatic Toxicology 11: 357-377, 1988.

34. GoVeg.com, "Health Concerns: Contamination" http://www.goveg.com/contamination.asp Accessed September 28, 2005.

35. Action PA, "Dioxin Homepage," http://www.ejnet.org/dioxin/#food Accessed September 22, 2005.

36. Fries, George F. "A Review of the Significance of Animal Food Products as Potential Pathways of Human Exposure to Dioxins," J. Anim. Sci. 73 (1995) 1639-1650.

37. Kogevinas, M., "Human health effects of dioxins: cancer, reproductive and endocrine system effects," Human Reproduction Update, Vol. 7 No. 3 (2001) 331-339.

38. Mandal, Prabir K., "Dioxin: a review of its environmental effects and its aryl hydrocarbon receptor biology," J Comp Physiol B 175 (2005) 221-230.

39. Charnley and Doull, "Human exposure to dioxins from food, 1999-2002," Food and Chemical Toxicology 43 (2005) 671-679.

40. Konishi, et al., "Continuous surveillance of organochlorine compounds in human breast milk from 1972 to 1998 in Osaka, Japan," Arch Environ Contam Toxicol 40 (2001) 571-578.

41. Baars, et al., "Dioxins, dioxin-like PCBs and non-dioxinlike PCBs in foodstuffs: occurrence and dietary intake in The Netherlands," Toxicology Letters 151 (2004) 51-61.

42. Kiviranta, et al., "Market basket study on dietary intake of PCDD/Fs, PCBs, and PBDEs in Finland," Environmental International 30 (2004) 923-932.

43. IARC (1990) as cited in Cole, et al., "Dioxin and cancer: a critical review," Regulatory Toxicology and Pharmacology, 38 (2003) pp. 378-388.

44. Wolfle and Marquardt, "Antioxidants inhibit the enhancement of malignant cell transformation induced by 2,3,7,8- tetrachlorodibenzo-p¬-dioxin," Carcinogenesis, Vol. 17 No. 6 (1996) 1273-1278.

45. Safe, et al., "Mechanisms of inhibitory aryl hydrocarbon receptor-estrogen receptor crosstalk in human breast cancer cells," J Mammary Gland Biol Neoplasia Vol. 5 No. 3 (2000) 295- 306.

46. Cole, et al., "Dioxin and cancer: a critical review," Regulatory Toxicology and Pharmacoogy 38 (2003) 378-388.

47. Kim and Milner, "Targets for indole-3-carbinol in cancer prevention," J Nutr Biochem Vol. 16 No. 2 (2005) 65-73.

48. Europa, "Environment: Chemical Accident Prevention, Preparedness and Response," http://europa.eu.int/comm environment/seveso/Accessed September 28, 2005.

49. Rolland, Rosalind M., "A review of chemically-induced alterations in thyroid and vitamin A status from field studies of wildlife and fish," Journal of Wildlife Diseases Vol. 36 No. 4 (2000) 615-635.

50. Safe and Krishnan, "Chlorinated hydrocarbons: estrogens and antiestrogens," Toxicol Lett 82-83 (1995) 731-6.

51. Blankenship et al., "Mechanisms of TCDD-induced abnormalities and embryo lethality in white leghorn chickens," Comparative Biochemistry and Physiology Part C 136 (2003) 47-62.

52. Wang et al., "Human dietary intake and excretion of dioxin-like compounds," J Environ Monit. Vol. 5 No. 2 (2003) 224-8.

53. Ryan and Patry, "Body burdens and exposure from food for polybrominated diphenyl ethers (BDEs) in Canada," The Second International Workshop on Brominated Flame Retardants, Stockholm May 14-16. Stolkholm, Sweden: Stockholm, University, 2001. p. 103. As cited in Kirivanta (2004) op cit.

54. Kokichi et al., "Fish intake plasma ?-3 polyunsaturated fatty acids, and polychlorinated dibenzo-p-dioxins/polychlorinated dibenzo-furans and co-planar polychlorinated biphenyls in the blood of the Japanese population," Int Arch Occup Environ Health (2003) 76: 205- 215.

55. Papadopoulos et al., "Levels of dioxins and dioxin-like PCBs in food samples on the Greek market," Chemosphere 57 (2004) 413-419.

56. US FDA, "Dioxin Analysis Results/Exposure Estimates," http://www.cfsan.fda.gov/~lrd/dioxdata.html Accessed September 27, 2005.

57. US FDA, "2003 TDS Dioxin Analysis: Summary," http://www.cfsan.fda.gov/September 27, 2005.

58. USDA, "USDA National Nutrient Database for Standard Reference, Release 17," http://www.nal.usda.gov/fnic/foodcomp/Data/SR17/wtrank/wt_rank.html Accessed September 27, 2005.

59. Schlummer et al., "Digestive tract absorption of PCDD/Fs, PCBs, and HCB in humans: mass balances and mechanistic considerations," Toxicology and Applied Pharmacology, 152 (1998) 128-137.

60. Aozasa, et al., "Fecal excretion of dioxin in mice enhanced by intake of dietary fiber bearing chlorophyllin," Bull. Environ. Contam. Toxicol. 70 (2003) 359-366.

61. Flesch-Janys, et al., "Elimination of polychlorinated dibenzo-p-dioxins and dibenzofurans in occupationally exposed persons," Journal of Toxicology and Environmental Health, 47 (1996) 363-378.

62. van der Plas, et al., "Effects of subchronic exposure to complex mixtures of dioxin-like and non-dioxin-like polyhalogenated aromatic compounds on thyroid hormone and vitamin A levels in female Sprague-Dawley rats," Toxicological Sciences 59 (2001) 92-100.

63. Lorick et al., "2,3,7,8-tetrachlorodibenzo-p-dioxin alters retinoic acid receptor function in human keratinocytes," Biochemical and Biophysical Research Communications, 243 (1998) 749-752.

64. Wang and Safe, "Interaction of 2,,7,8-tetrachlorodibenzo-p-dioxin and retinoic acid in MCF-7 human breast cancer cells," Toxicology and Applied Pharmacology, 127 (1994) 1-8.

65. Yang et al., "Inhibitory effects of vitamin A on TCDD-induced cytochrome P-450 1A1 enzyme activity and expression," Toxicological Sciences, Vol. 85 No. 1 (2005) 727-734.

66. Livera, et al., "Regulation and perturbation of testicular functions by vitamin A," Reproduction 124 (2002) 173-180.

67. World Health Organization, "Vitamin A deficiency," http://www.who.int/nut/vad.htm Accessed September 28, 2005.

68. The Merck Manual, "Vitamin A deficiency," http://www.merck.com/mrkshared/mmanual/ section1/ chapter3/3b.jsp Accessed September 28, 2005.

69. Fallon and Enig, "Vitamin A Saga," http://www.westonaprice.org/basicnutrition/vitaminasaga.html Accessed September 28, 2005.

70. Harvey et al., Biochemistry: 3rd Edition, Baltimore: Lippincott Williams and Williams (2005) 382.

71. Fletcher, et al., "Hepatic vitamin A depletion is a sensitive marker of 2,3,7,8-tetrachlorodibenzo- p¬-dioxin (TCDD) exposure in four rodent species," Toxicological Sciences 62 (2001) 166-175.

72. Fiorella, et al., "2,3,7,8-tetrachlorodibenzo-p-dioxin induces diverse retinoic acid metabolites in multiple tissues of the Sprague-Dawley rat," Toxicology and Applied Pharmacology, 134 (1995) 222-228.

73. Stohs, et al., "Effects of BHA, d-alpha-tocopherol and retinol acetate on TCDD-mediated changes in lipid peroxidation, glutathione peroxidase activity and survival," Xenobiotica Vol. 14 No. 7 (1984) 533-7.

74. Alsharif, et al., "Protective effects of vitamin A and vitamin E succinate against 2,3,7,8-tetrachlorodibenzo-p¬-dioxin (TCDD)-induced body wasting, hepatomegaly, thymic atrophy, production of reactive oxygen species and DNA damage in C57Bl/6J mice," Basic and Clinical Pharmacology and Toxicology 95 (2004) 131-138.

75. "Free Radical Introduction" http://www.exrx.net/Nutrition/Antioxidants/Introduction.html Accessed September 27, 2005.

76. Linus Pauling Institute's Micronutrient Information Center, "Coenzyme Q10," http://lpi.oregonstate.edu/infocenter/othernuts/coq10/index.html Accessed September 27, 2005.

77. Linus Pauling Institute's Micronutrient Information Center, "Vitamin C," http://lpi.oregonstate.edu/infocenter/vitamins/vitaminC/index.html Accessed September 27, 2007.

78. Hilscherova, et al., "Oxidative stress in liver and brain of the hatchling chicken (Gallus domesticus) following in ovo injection with TCDD," Comparative Biochemistry and Physiology Part C 136 (2003) 29-45.

79. Chelchowska, et al., "Lipids and vitamin A and E status in vegetarian children," Med Wieku Rozwoj, 7 (2003) 577-585.

80. Kovacikova, "Antioxidant status in vegetarians and nonvegetarians in Bratislava region," Z Ernahrungswiss, Vol. 37 No. 2 (1998) 178-182.

81. Bederova, et al., "Comparison of nutrient intake and corresponding biochemical parameters in adolescent vegetarians and non-vegetarians," Cas Lek Cesk. Vol. 139 No. 13 (2000) 396- 400.

82. Smith, "Dietary Supplementation of vitamin E to cattle to improve shelf life and case life of beef for domestic and international markets," Colorado State University, Fort Collins, Colorado 80523-1171 as cited in Eat Wild, "Nutritional Benefits of Grassfarming," http://www.eatwild.com/nutrition.html Accessed September 27, 2005.

83. West et al., "Consequences of revised estimates of carotenoid bioefficacy for dietary control of vitamin A deficiency in developing countries," J. Nutr. Vol 132 No. 9 Suppl. (2002) 2920S-2926S.

84. Tang et al., "Short-term (intestinal) and long-term (post-intestinal) conversion of beta-carotene to retinol in adults as assessed by a stable-isotope reference method," Am J ClinNutr, Vol. 8 No. 2 (2003) 259-266.

85. Ohtake, et al., "Effects of dietary lipids on daunomycin-induced nephropathy in mice: comparison between cod liver oil and soybean oil," Lipids, Vol. 37 No. 4 (2002) 359-366.

86. Diniz, et al., "Diets rich in saturated and polyunsaturated fatty acids: metabolic shifting and cardiac health," Nutrition, 200 (2004) 230-234.

87. Saito and Kubo, "Relationship between tissue lipid peroxidation and peroxidizability index after a-linolenic, eicosapentaenoic, or docosahexaenoic acid intake in rats," British Journal of Nutrition, 89 (2003) 19-28.

88. Hunkar, et al., "Effects of cod liver oil on tissue antioxidant pathways in normal and streptozotocin-diabetic rats," Cell Biochem Funct. Vol. 20 No. 4 (2002) 297-302.

89. Enig, Mary G. and Sally Fallon, "Tripping Lightly Down the Prostaglandin Pathways," http://www.westonaprice.org/knowyourfats/tripping.html Accessed September 28, 2005.

90. Sears M.D., Al, The Doctor's Heart Cure, St. Paul: Dragon Door (2004) 136-143.

91. Fraps, G. S. & Meinke, W. W. (1945) Arch. Biochem., 6, 323 as cited in World Health Organization, International Programme [sic] on Chemical Safety, "Toxicological evlautation of some food colours, enzymes, flavour enhancers, thickening agents, and certain food additives," http://www.inchem.org/documents/jecfa/jecmono/v06je15.htm Accessed October 2, 2007.

92. Price, Weston A., Nutrition and Physical Degeneration: 6th Edition, La Mesa: Price Pottenger Nutrition Foundation (2000) 293.

Other Books By Benita and Jim

Other Books By Benita and Jim

Renewal

Feeling stressed? Anxious? Nervous? Learn what behaviors can feed stress and how to change these behaviors to reduce it. Learn stress management and the best ways to deal with panic attacks. Find other resources to help you cope with anxiety. ISBN # 978-1440413347

Put Your Weight Loss in Overdrive

Do you want to lose weight? Are you willing to eat healthier and make changes in your diet? If you are willing to follow our lead and replace your unhealthy diet with even some of the super foods we tell you about in this book, you will put your diet in overdrive. Weight loss will be a snap. We guarantee it. This book makes weight loss easy. ISBN # 978-1440413320

Life Management

Are you organized? Then you aren't the person we're looking for. If you aren't as organized as you think you should be, this is the book for you. Say goodbye to clutter and let order reign. We provide clever home and family management tips.; time saving tips and more. Get help managing your life. ISBN # 978-1440417458

You Want It When?

Are you a procrastinator? Do you put off doing things until just before they're due? Do you do your Christmas shopping on Christmas Eve? There is help for all of you right here. Learn how to break the procrastination habit.
ISBN # 978-1440417067

ABC's of Goal Setting

Ever set goals and write them down? What happened? Did you reach any of them or did you give up before you got there? Supercharge your goal setting and get ready for that satisfaction that only comes after reaching one of your goals. This book makes goal setting easy.
ISBN # 978-1440419183

An Introduction To Traditional Chinese Medicine

Tired of prescriptions? of taking hundreds of pills? You've probably wondered about acupuncture and chinese medicine but were afraid to take the plunge without knowing just a little bit more about what is involved and how it could benefit you. In *An Introduction To Traditional Chinese Medicine*, Benita and Jim will explain how Acupuncture, Yoga and Qigong can help you attain and stay healthy and what system of beliefs are behind how they work.
ISBN # 978-1440424586

Coming Soon

You Were Born To Excel

This book is based on a series of classes we compiled back in June of 1998. The classes were called Human Excellence Engineering. The basic series consisted of six classes as presented in this book. Two to three weeks were spent on each class. An advanced series was planned and begun but never completed. The topics covered are: In chapter 1: New Thinking Skills; in chapter 2: Inside You; in chapter 3: Changing the Past; in chapter 4: A Brighter Today; in chapter 5: Feeling Good Again; and in chapter 6: The Future Begins Here. The classes and hence, the material in this book are a combination of NLP, Psychology and Shamanism. ISBN # (not yet assigned)

Personal Trance-formations

More than ever, researchers are concerned with the effects of mental and emotional states on an individuals health and with the possibility of treating the patient as an active and responsible participant in the healing process rather than as a passive recipient of either the disease or the cure.

It is this emphasis that provides the basis for using a variety of techniques that enable non-medical persons to control pain perception and create their own response to illness. The mind plays a vital role in healing, more even than modern medicine has so far acknowledged. This guidebook to your inner world, the inner landscape of your soul, will help you connect with your most authentic feelings and thoughts. It contains a variety of techniques for dealing with this deep inner material. ISBN # (not yet assigned)

Approaching Wisdom

Storytelling is essential to the shaman's craft. There was more to the old tales than just a good yarn. Woven into the thrills and emotions were messages. The tales are the framework of the lore and the lore is a body of teachings and an essential part of the shaman's working life. Through lore we re- create the ancient strands of Otherworldly knowledge buried deep in our unconscious and bring them to the forefront of our conscious mind. We can then see them from a new perspective and apply them to life in our "everyday" world. This book recreates the shaman's storytelling as a quest for wisdom. In it we explore ways through story, myth and exercises to expand your sensory awareness, achieve internal union and contact your transpersonal self. This book provides tools, but the real exploration is up to you. ISBN # (not yet assigned)

The Castle of the Grail

The Quest for the Grail is not a fairy tale for children. It is a serious undertaking. The journey is full of trials and tribulations. The inner landscape of the Quest is full of dark forests, winding paths, narrow places, bridges, gates and castles. It is a very confusing place for us because we start foolish and ignorant. We do not recognize our guide and are frightened of what we might find. We are tested severely and ruthlessly but with mercy. The Quest is about Self Transformation and personal liberation. There is a unifying principle at the heart of all of these ways of thought, which can only be grasped by symbols, analogies and myths. Jung explained this with his archetypes of the collective unconscious.
ISBN # (not yet assigned)

The Gold Mine in PLR.

What is PLR? How can it benefit you? P.L. and R. are the initial letters of Private Label Rights. PLR is merchandise or software, most of which is info or text based, customizable, and reusable as your own. The concept of PLR differs only slightly from having a ghostwriter. So if you have a website and need fresh content or are a writer and need fresh ideas - this book is a must have! ISBN # (not yet assigned)

Creativity

Would you like to be more creative? More intuitive? Would you like to learn creative problem solving? You can with the proper training. You probably already are intuitive and creative without realizing it. This book will provide the training you need to handle anything life throws at you in a more creative way. ISBN # (not yet assigned)

Never Pay for Computer Software Again

Would you like to get a totally free operating system for your PC? How about an office suite that is rated better than Microsoft Office without Microsoft's price tag? Would you like free Image manipulation (Graphics) software? Games, Productivity software, Business applications - and all for free? How about one of the best web browsers around? Interested? It's all explained right here in Never Pay for Computer Software Again. Interested? You should be. ISBN # (not yet assigned)

Surviving Life

How do you stay cheerful in the face of adversity, loss of job, bankruptcy, taxes and all the other things that life can throw at you? ISBN # (not yet assigned)

(It's Your Book) Take Control

Covers everything the author needs to know about self publishing. Copyrights, ISBN numbers, writing software versus page layout software, cover design, book layout, POD versus conventional printing methods, marketing, distribution, advertising, etc. ISBN # (not yet assigned)

The Family Book of Fairy Tales

Stories of Princes and Princess's, enchanted giants and mighty ogres, lions, tailors and onions collected from around the world and assembled in this book to amuse you and your children. Includes the following stories: Cinderella's Daughter, The Giant's Hand, The Prince and the Lions, The Three Buns, The Boyer's Bride, How the Sea Became Salt, The Captive Princess, The Enchanted Oranges, The Knight of the Onion Shield, The Trade That No One Knew and The Prince and The Tailor. ISBN # 978-1441435057

Benita's Encyclopedia of Crystals and Stones

What gems, crystals or stones have healing properties? Which do not? Which stones would you use for High Blood Pressure? Which for blood disorders? Which stones would be more effective for sores and wounds? How would you use Calcite in healing? ISBN # (not yet assigned)

Handy Order Form

Fax orders: 520-297-1293. (Send this form)

Telephone orders: 520-297-1293 Have your credit card handy.

Email orders: Tranzform@Comcast.net <Attn. Orders>

Postal orders: Orders * 8571 N. Calle Tioga * Oro Valley, Az. 85704

Please send the following books, software or reports. I understand that I may return any of them for a full refund for any reason.

ISBN No. _____   Quantity ☐

Title: _____

ISBN No. _____   Quantity ☐

Title: _____

Name: _____

Address:_____

City: _____   State : _____   Zip: _____

Phone:
_____

Email: _____

I would like more information on other books   ☐
and/ or products

Arizona residents: Please add 8.1% Sales Tax

Handy Order Form

Fax orders: 520-297-1293. (Send this form)

Telephone orders: 520-297-1293 Have your credit card handy.

Email orders: Tranzform@Comcast.net <Attn. Orders>

Postal orders: Orders * 8571 N. Calle Tioga * Oro Valley, Az. 85704

Please send the following books, software or reports. I understand that I may return any of them for a full refund for any reason.

ISBN No. _____ Quantity [   ]

      Title: _____

ISBN No. _____ Quantity [   ]

      Title: _____

Name: _____

Address: _____

City: _____ State : _____ Zip: _____

Phone:
    _____

Email: _____

I would like more information on other books
and/ or products   [   ]

Arizona residents: Please add 8.1% Sales Tax